INTERDEPENDENCE:
The Route to Community
Second Edition

INTERDEPENDENCE:
The Route to Community
Second Edition

Al Condeluci, Ph.D.
Executive Director, UCP Centre for Personal
Development

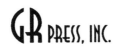

GR PRESS, INC.

Revised edition.
© 1995 by GR Press, Inc
 PO Box 4116
Winter Park, Florida 32793-4116
(800) 438-5911

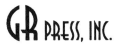

Originally published by PMD Press, Inc. © 1991.

ISBN: 1-878205-11-0
Library of Congress Catalog Card Number: 91-72030

Printed in the United States of America

Dedication

***To Sinbad and Jane Condeluci, my parents, guides, and friends
You set the stage for all of this***

CONTENTS

Preface to the Second Edition

Preface to the Second Edition

It's amazing to me the impact we can make on people and not even know it. There are countless people that we come in contact with who might hear what we say or see what we do and change their behavior. We humans serve as models and look for guides all the time. It's not only how we learn and adopt new behaviors, but also how our culture comes to evolve.

Over and above all this is the influence that comes with the written word. Through books, articles, newspapers, and magazines we come to develop, forge, reinforce, or change ideas. I remember reading an article a few years ago where the author had asked a number of knowledgeable and influential people to identify the five books that had the greatest impact on them. Now stop for a minute and reflect on this. How would you answer this question?

Such is the power of the written word and anyone who takes pen to paper for the purpose of sharing new ideas or influencing thought must appreciate this power. I was humbled in this thought recently when I received a letter from a person in the state of Washington who had just finished reading *Interdependence* and felt compelled to write. His was a warm and kind letter that told me he was led to *Interdependence* by a friend who told him it was a "must read." It was nice to learn of this, but for me it also drove home the seriousness and importance of the impact of the written word.

Since the publication of *Interdependence*, I have been encouraged by the interest and debate it has stirred. Over these years, I have visited most every state in the United States and every providence in Canada. I have conducted hundreds of workshops and retreats and countless speeches and presentations. All of these efforts have continued to validate the usefulness of *Interdependence* as a conceptual framework for understanding and, more importantly, adjusting the way we come to know and support people who have some type of difference that has caused them to be stigmatized.

Currently, we are in the throes of dilemma in rehabilitation. Although technology is advancing, the social state for most people with severe disabilities remains challenging. In spite of all the "new" rehabilitative approaches, people with disabling conditions are still caught up in the same traditional stereotypes and mental models. People are still devalued and institutionalized at a drop of a hat. Indeed, the most advanced federal funding opportunities for people with disabilities to stay in the community, Title XIX, is still designated as a wavier. Know that a "waiver" is an exception to the rule, and the current rule for Title XIX funding is institutionalization.

The job market opportunities are not better. According to the most recent Louis Harris Poll (1994), people with disabilities are the most unemployed and underemployed segment in America.

Even though these situations are bad, what is most troubling is that people with severe disabilities are not active or involved in the clubs, groups, and associations of our culture. Stop for a moment and think about these venues in your life. Think about the clubs, groups, and associations you belong to — the PTA's, YMCA's, church groups, reading clubs, fraternal, or service organizations. Now think about the membership of these groups. How many people with severe disabilities are present in these groups that you attend? I know for me, there are a scant few.

Now, why is it, that in spite of our best intentions, efforts, and actions, so many people with severe disabilities are so far removed from the typical venues of our culture? Why haven't we done better? What continues to hold us back?

All of these questions are examined in *Interdependence*. The book explores the reasons why people are disempowered, the paradigms that currently encase rehabilitation and a review of our community today. Additionally, *Interdependence* outlines a new paradigm for human services and articulates ways this paradigm can be achieved.

Know, however, that this thesis has not always been that welcomed in the rehabilitation field. Because *Interdependence* challenges the existing medical paradigm, it has frightened or angered some people. It is important to know that paradigms root deeply and when a paradigm that you have grown up around is challenged, the natural reaction is to become defensive and angry. And so a debate has followed. Regardless of where people stand on the question — Is rehabilitation successful in helping people return to the community? — at the least, *Interdependence* is getting people to talk. This discussion is vital to not only the future of rehabilitation, but to the evolution of our culture and community as well.

This second edition of *Interdependence* is, by large, unchanged from its 1991 version. Along with this new preface, Chapter 5 has been redone and retitled, "Understanding Culture and the Community." Here, we look more closely at the basic notion of community and culture as the primary point of impact for rehabilitation or any other type of service designed for people who have been devalued. I have also added an epilogue that outlines some segue points for consideration before taking a look at my second book, *Beyond Difference*. This work, second in a trilogy I have prepared in understanding *Interdependence*, is an inward exploration. If you find *Interdependence* helpful or provocative, I hope you will consider reading *Beyond Difference* as well.

Before I close this preface, I have another thought to share. This has to do with the isolated nature of writing. That is, as a person who enjoys being around or with others people, writing tends to be a lonely exercise. One sits with their thoughts and assembles them into a thesis, commits them to paper and then waits for reaction to their writings. Although I have done this with *Interdependence*, I am more used to talking face to face where one can read reactions and respond immediately. Further, if the writings are controversial, as some claim *Interdependence* to be, then the gap is even greater.

To adjust for this isolation, I am asking you to make *Interdependence* an interactive tool. As you read it, mark it up. You'll notice that we have designed it with margins for just this purpose. If you find parts controversial, scribble in your thoughts. Why do you feel as you do?

What might you do about how change could be made? Then, after you have really mixed it up with the book, turn to the very end and notice my address. Take a minute to drop me a note and let me know your thoughts. Not only will this help you to focus your thoughts, but it will also help a lonely writer get the feedback he needs.

So thanks for selecting *Interdependence* as your next read. I hope you find it to be helpful.

Al Condeluci
McKees Rocks, PA
October, 1994

Preface

I invent nothing.
I rediscover.

Auguste Rodin

Preface

This work is a synthesis. That is why Rodin's quote is such a
good starting point. Over my 20 years in human services, I have
been hunting and searching. I entered the human service field
at an exciting time, the late 60s, as an undergraduate student
at Youngstown State University. Intrigued by human behavior
and driven by the broader ideas to better the world, I made my
way. First, as an orphanage volunteer, and then after gradua-
tion with a larger geriatric hospital. In 1973, I moved to a
community based agency focused on disability issues. In
between, and along the way I continued formal studies at the
University of Pittsburgh.

In this journey, I have met many people, read many books,
attended many conferences, and heard many speeches. I have
related with thousands of agency representatives, spent time
with countless people with disabilities and families, and scores
of public officials. I have been a student and a teacher, a giver
and a taker, a thinker and a doer. I have researched, written,
defended, and critiqued. I have been in front and behind. Most
of all, I have thought.

In a way, this book is a reflection of this journey. It is an
amalgamation of many thoughts, ideas, and innovations. Some
come from the great thinkers, those that have literally revolu-
tionized their fields. Other ideas come from simple folks, ones
that are not found in the literature; from common people who

are struggling, or have struggled and have learned from the experience.

As I have found, heard, or read these ideas, I have taken the ones that seem to fit my reality and have organized them into a flow that works for me. In this organization, I have had opportunity to share and discuss them with friends and associates around the United States and Canada. In this effort, others have found my synthesis to make sense to them as well. I was invited to share more and then to write.

And so, what you have in front of you is a humble effort to capture and organize these thoughts and ideas. I have woven them in a way that fits for me. Written in a style that is natural for me. To this extent, you are not getting the typical, academic perspective, but a more folksy blend of ideas and stories. I have referenced specific authors and their work, as well as identified important passages from their work. Still, I see this book as an informal reflection on a vexing challenge. I have written it in a way that I hope appeals to all of us who relate to people who have been devalued or disenfranchised.

Any man who afflicts the human race with ideas must be prepared to see them misunderstood.

H.L. Mencken

Interdependence is about relationships. It is a composite blend of a number of viable concepts into a rational approach to the human elements of devaluation. Built from the works of sociologists, systems analysts, educators, organizers, urban planners, psychologists, politicians, academicians and some common folk, interdependence attempts to make practical sense out of our current state for people who are disenfranchised from society. Despite some academic components, interdependence is, in essence, a simple concept; one that subscribes more to the wisdom of common sense and plain speaking. In a best case scenario, it applies and integrates theoretical concepts into an approach that is basic to understand and utilize.

In this book, I use the term *interdependence* in a number of ways. It is important for the reader to understand, however, that the term relates to an approach, a way of relating to people who have been devalued or disenfranchised. When I say things such as, "Interdependence mandates that we connect people to communities," I am suggesting that the approach be that people are connected. Another way of understanding the word's use is as a fulcrum for action. Interdependence is a model, movement, and paradigm to link people who have been disenfranchised from their community.

By disenfranchisement, I am referring to the process whereby a person or group of persons become distanced or ostracized from society or their community. Although disenfranchisement can be self-oriented, more often than not, it is a distantiation levied by society toward the individual. In most cases, the disenfranchisement is caused by some difference or distinction of the individual that is alien or misunderstood by society. This difference can be a number of things, but usually is something that is devalued. That is, the difference is something that is not sought out by the majority of people as being worthwhile or desirable. Examples of these differences can be age, illness, physical disabilities, intelligence, race, religion, income, or skill. Interdependence is about a reunion of these distanced people to their community.

Recently, I had the opportunity to review a report on self-esteem, prepared by the California Task Force to Promote Self-Esteem and Personal and Social Responsibility. The report, titled *Toward a State of Esteem* (1990) recognized the generic importance of interdependence. They stated, "We act responsibly when we encourage people to grow beyond dependence toward independence and interdependence." Further, they recognized the vital importance of self-esteem in the empowerment process of people who have been offset from community. Specifically, they identify five areas that make people particularly vulnerable. These groups are:

1. Aging
2. AIDS
3. Hunger and Homelessness
4. Physical Disability
5. Racism

Similarly, *Interdependence* reaches out to these same "at risk" areas. Although examples and strategies utilized in this work came from a disability perspective, I believe the concept fits well with any distantiated group.

All information is imperfect,
we have to treat it with humility.

J. Bronowski

Oriental culture speaks to a concept called *shibumi.* This word refers to something that is both simple and complex at the same time. A good example of *shibumi* would be the reality of a Japanese garden. When you come upon a Japanese garden you might be struck by its simplicity. The rocks and streams coupled with the bonsai trees make for a basic scene. Yet, looking closer, you may begin to notice the detail of its beauty. The rocks are just so and the bonsai tree is trimmed to accentuate the flow of the stream and you then recognize the complexity of its reality. The garden is indeed *shibumi.*

To a certain extent, the concept of interdependence could be considered the same way. As stated earlier, interdependence is about relationships; a person's relationship with others, their focal community, and their greater community. A quick analysis might point to the simplicity of this concept. People relating with other people is a basic interchange. Yet, when considering the situation of individuals who have been systematically disenfranchised from their community, for whatever reason, the idea of relationship development takes on a whole new perspective. The reasons for why one is disenfranchised, how it relates to devaluation, and the effects that this disenfranchisement has on how the community sees them, and more importantly, how they see themselves are all complex factors that need to be considered. In this way, the basic concept of relating and making friends must be tempered off the complexity of the factors that have led to their devaluation.

In spite of these complexities, the concept of interdependence is a movement back to basics. That is, in the advent of human services in the United States and Canada (and in most other industrialized countries) there has been a propensity to overspecialize the deviance factors of those who have been disenfranchised. Although there are clear reasons why this phenomena has occurred, the march of specialization has been steady and powerful. In the case of disability alone, there was a time when people with disabilities were a part of the community. Regardless of their skills and abilities. These folks were a part of their neighborhood and accepted as such. Then, with the development of rehabilitation as a medical specialty, human service workers felt that these people with disabilities might be better treated (from both a medical and quality of life sense) if they were in environments that the experts could develop and control. Thus, a form of institutionalization was forced.

This concept of institutionalization is important to an understanding of interdependence. In his book, *Asylums*, Erving Goffman (1961), defines an institution to be:

> . . . *a place of residence and work where a large number of like-situated individuals, cut off from the wider society for an appreciable period of time, together lead an enclosed, formally administered round of life.*

Without question, many disenfranchised groups have been relegated to institutional settings. Some because they are a threat to society, others because it was felt that such settings were the most beneficial or therapeutic for the different individual.

Now, I have no basic quarrel with the intent of those at the root of this action. I am sure they were concerned people and that they wanted to make things better for people with disabilities. I do, however, quarrel with the approach and bold thrust of specialization, especially when this approach can create far greater problems of disenfranchisement for those very people the experts intended to help.

In the early 30s, Ortega y Gasset wrote about the "barbarism of specialization." His concern was that specialization might lead to an insensitivity with people focusing on only one dimension. This caution, I believe, is still instructive today.

Interdependence attempts to overview this phenomena and to offer other thoughts and approaches to the problem of disenfranchisement and reconnection. In a spirit of *shibumi*, it acknowledges complexity, but unlike previous reviews, it looks not at complexity of the person who has been disenfranchised. Rather, it looks at the complexities of societal reactions to devaluation. Quite simply, it suggests that it is not the person, but society's perspective of the person that needs to be addressed.

This critical differentiation is vital to understanding *Interdependence*. Keep in mind that for years the experts have been struggling to look deeper and deeper into the problems and deficits of those considered to be different. They have analyzed and reanalyzed these deficits. The problems of the disenfranchised have been labeled and recorded in the professional journals, taught in the universities, and publicized in the mass media. Most of us know well the problems and deficits of the major maladies of society.

I believe, and *Interdependence* attempts to describe, that this energy and approach has been misguided. This propensity to articulate what is wrong with people is one of the very reasons why these same people remain disenfranchised. Further, this theory concludes that in the zeal of human services to help those with challenges it has, in essence, perpetuated more problems. Indeed, in some cases, it has made things worse for the very people it wants to help.

Ideas are tools — you can play with them, turn them around, look at them, use and test them.

Myles Horton

In his seminal work, *Medial Nemesis*, Ivan Illich (1976), articulated the concept of iatrogensis. In a review of medicine, he concluded that in many regards the physician caused more harm than good. The term *iatrogenic* means just that; physician-created harm. The concept of interdependence inspects iatrogensis on a broader scale. For many, disenfranchised people, harm is created or levied on them not necessarily by physicians, but by socially sanctioned human service workers. This phenomena of iatrogenisis is explored at greater length later in this book.

A recognition of these complexities, however, leads way to a new commitment to the simplicity of relationships. After all the cards are cut, for most of us, quality of life boils down to commitments and relationships, people to people, and one to one. *Interdependence* is a work that recognizes this fact and suggests a paradigm shift for those organizations, advocates, family, and friends who care about reuniting the disenfranchised. It offers an understanding of what might have gone askew in our zeal to help. It focuses on how these approaches can and do create harm. More importantly it poses ideas and thoughts for change.

As a synthesis, *Interdependence* builds on past works and weaves current material together to create a sense of the issues of today. To this extent, I am indebted to those thinkers, past and present, who laid the groundwork for this thesis. Without their bold and often provocative works, a text such as *Interdependence* could not have been produced.

In writing this book I have attempted to weave the concepts that surround devaluation with stories and thoughts from my experiences and those that have happened to my friends. The good fortune I have had to travel and share ideas with people around the United States and Canada have been essential to this thrust. In this effort, I have done my best to portray groups and situations as fairly and accurately as possible. My sensitivity however, has been tempered with attempting to make my points and if at any point I have misrepresented a group, or have used inappropriate terminology, I beg your forgiveness. For example, at times I have used the pronoun "his" as a description. This is done purely to help the text to flow and to avoid awkward terms such as "his/her." To this extent, I thank you for this indulgence.

This work starts with a look at the phenomena of disempowerment. Issues such as oppression, role formation, stereotypes, imaging, other movements, the independent living movement, and the nature of rehabilitation are all explored and woven together to create a theme.

Next, the text turns to examine the four major paradigms that relate to or influence human services today. These include, the medical paradigm, the educational paradigm, the economic paradigm, and the maintenance paradigm. Each are analyzed via the perceived problem, core, actions, power base, and goals. Additionally, an overview of human service settings today is reported.

The third section of the text introduces the interdependent paradigm for human services and presents its key features. Here, essential elements are described and the basic steps to application are introduced. As success in interdependence depends on a natural reintegration to community, these four elements and community becomes vital to the next sections of the text.

In the fourth chapter, the book turns to achieving interdependence. The four component parts essential to interdependence, role competency, supplemental supports, bridge-building, and systems advocacy, are explored and detailed. Practical examples and suggestions are reviewed.

In the fifth section, the concept of culture and community is defined and discussed. It is amazing how little our present human services know about community. Given this void, Interdependence articulates community features and the important aspects of understanding the formal and informal systems.

A final concluding chapter pulls it all together. Suggestions are made as to how interdependence relates to all types of groups that are disenfranchised.

Last is an epilogue to this second edition. It is a personal afterword to update the reader.

Interdependence is an important work. Although it examines some negative things, it is hopeful that a paradigm shift from the expert oriented paradigms presently dominating human services will give way to interdependence. That people presently oppressed, wounded, and in some cases at serious risk through present practices, will not only be empowered, but will rise to a level of interrelationships. This text works hard to promote such shifting.

There is a revolution coming. It will not be like revolutions of the past. It will originate with the individual and with culture, and it will change the political structure only in its final act. It will not require violence to succeed, and it can not be successfully resisted by violence . . . it promises a higher reason, a more human community, and a new and liberated individual.

Charles Reich

Acknowledgments

Acknowledgments

In 1978, I was invited to join a national faculty pulled together by the Federal Department of Housing and Urban Development. Our project, titled "Handi-TAP," was designed to provide guidance and stimulation to local private and public agencies interested in housing for people with disabilities. As my agency, United Cerebral Palsy of Pittsburgh, has been a national leader in developing and implementing creative housing support systems for people with disabilities since 1973, it was felt we could contribute solid ideas and strategies.

The "Handi-TAP" project (Handicap-Technical Assistance Project) operated over the next two years bringing its message to 20 cities around the United States. I had the good fortune to participate in most of these gatherings. I acknowledge this experience because for me it was my first challenge to articulate the embryonic concepts of interdependence. In a public way, an idea was hatched.

Prior to my participation with the "Handi-TAP" project, like most other human service practitioners, I was busy trying to design and implement a residential support system that could work for people. I had been exposed to Wolf Wolfensberger's normalization principle and its effects in Canada, Nebraska and other parts of Pennsylvania. I also had the opportunity to learn the independent living concepts from Ed Roberts and his colleagues who ran Centers for Independent Living. Using both of these basic streams, normalization and the independent living philosophy, we had forged an interesting service delivery design in Pittsburgh.

"Handi-TAP" presented a real challenge to me in that at that point we had not really wrote about, or spoke out publicly on our service or the philosophy. When called forth by HUD to do this, I was pushed to a higher dimension. That is, in order to be a viable teacher, I felt compelled to be as articulate on our philosophy and service as possible. This led to further study, reading, dialogue, and introspection. Of course, this also led the way to wanting to know and aspire to more.

And so, as I move forward to introduce you to the concept of interdependence, it is only appropriate that I think about, acknowledge, and thank those who invited me, inspired me, and confronted me and the first to do that were my colleagues associated with "Handi-TAP." So thank you, Tom Urban, Betty Shaw, David Williams, Katherine Janka, David Lipsey, Mary Ann Allard, David Evans, and the others involved in this project. Of course there have been many other experiences prior to and since "Handi-TAP." I would be remiss if I didn't point them out. Since I feel my experiences in developing *Interdependence* have come in eras and waves, it is easiest for me to acknowledge people this way. So here they are:

UCP Influences

Thanks to Fred Enck, my mentor and partner since 1973. Others equally close to my growth are: Sharon Gretz, Jan Bayfield, Darla Lynn, Mary Lou Busby, Judy Weiss, Bob Mochan, Mike Beachler, Jay Carson, Rick Boyle, Bill McDowell, Sue Dietz, Tom Kearney, Ray Smith, Jim Prentice, Rich Hubert, Harry White, and many more folks too numerous to name here. Administrative supports include: Edie Scales, Nancy Collins and Laverne Walton. A special thinks to Carol Litzinger, my principal typist and support person. Carol did yeoman work to pound out drafts, make valuable suggestions, and keep me encouraged.

Independent Living Influences

Over the years, I have had opportunity to meet and dialogue with many people about the concepts of choice and control. Some of these folks are: Ed Roberts, Fred Fay, Judy Heumann, Lex Friedan, Gini Laurie, Judy Barricella, Sigi Shapiro, Bill Chrisner, Nancy Jochiem, Gerben DeJong, Mark Johnson, Justin Dart, Nick Pagano, Kevin Capp, Keith Donati, Ruth Shannon, Lucy Spruill, and Clark Ross.

Normalization and Developmental Disabilities Influences

Although the principle of normalization (now known as Social Role Valorization) is separate from developmental disabilities, most of the people I have related to in this area embrace the concept. To this extent I have combined these categories. Thanks to: Guy Caruso, Thomas Neuville, Allen Bergmann, Jim Hollalhan, Michael Morris, Darcy Elks Miller, David Schwartz, Bob Garrett, Elmer Cerano, Gerry Provencal, Chuck Peters, John Ligato, Mel Knowlton, Dennis Felty, A.J. Hildebrand, Dianna Ploof, Susan Maczka, Thomas Gilhool, Steve Taylor, Henry Schwartz, Mark Murphy, Hank Bersani, Richard Rosenberg, and Jim O'Connor.

Head Injury Rehabilitation Influences

Since 1983, I have been involved in rehabilitation efforts for people with head injuries. This experience has been both formal and informal and is probably the most focused influence in the articulation of *Interdependence*. It has provided me with the opportunity to gain an international perspective and interchange with people from all over North America. Indeed, this exposure has led directly to the publication of articles, chapters, and this book. Thanks to: Pat Price, Marilyn Spivak, Gerry Bush, Janet Williams, Jean Bush, Dan Keating, Steve Vander-Schaff, Tim McCarron, Cheryl Palmer, Beth O'Brien-Causey, Jerid Fisher, Paul Spanbock, Mike McCue, Larry Doperak, John Pistorius, Andrea Bogden, Pete Swales, Pat DiPrima, Sheridan Barnes, Kenny Hosak, Sandy Milton, Ray Remple, John Simpson, David Seaton, Harvey Jacobs, Corky Boak, Barry Rather, Carl Stanko, Andre Dume, and many others too numerous to mention.

Equally, I appreciate the support and liberties offered by my publisher, GR Press, Inc. It was Paul Deutsch who urged me to prepare this book and I thank him for the confidence in my message and writing. Deep thanks too, to the editorial staff. Our many conversations and ideas were most helpful.

Finally, I save the most important acknowledgment for last. This book could not have happened if it was not for the most flexible and supportive family I know, mine. My wife, Liz was always available, to read passages, offer a tip, or simply help me spell a word; not to mention the overload of children duties while Daddy sat behind the word processor. And for children, in spite of their tender ages, my three were tremendously supportive. Thanks to Dante, Gianna and Santino. Your forgiveness for Daddy time lost is a lesson for us all.

As I close this acknowledgment section, I feel somewhat ambivalent. I have just rattled off many names of people I know, have spent time with in discussing concepts, or have helped me understand themes related to interdependence, yet that does not seem to be enough. How does one adequately acknowledge a culmination of thinking, ideas, discussions, and concepts that lead to a gestalt such as interdependence?

To those mentioned and the many who are not, please accept my thanks. In a humble way I hope *Interdependence* will help.

Al Condeluci
McKees Rocks, PA
February 1991

Introduction:
Stories From The Field

God will us free,
Man wills us slaves

D. Bliss, 1773

Introduction:
Stories From The Field

On a warm, fall day a few years ago, I drove from Pittsburgh, PA to Harrisburg, PA, the state capitol. I was with two friends and the purpose of our trip was to testify before a state human service committee.

After the long, four-hour trip, we arrived at our prearranged hotel and checked in. We were glad to be there and decided to get a quick drink in the lounge before we retired for the night.

The lounge was like most other hotel night spots, with a smattering of patrons spread here and there. We found a table and sat down, waiting for the waitress to take our order. In due time, she appeared and we made our orders. I asked for a beer, my friend Tom, a whiskey sour, and Harry a gin and tonic.

After what seemed like an eternity, she returned with an empty tray. She said, "I'm sorry, but I can't serve you."

"What's the problem, do you need to see cards?" I said fumbling for my wallet. "No," she said, looking nervous, "It's not cards," and she started to leave.

I ran after her, and asked, "Ma'am, what's the problem? Do we need to order food to get a drink?" She said, "You'll have to talk to the bartender," and hurried off. She looked and acted just like my mother had told me people look when they know they are in the wrong.

I went to the bar and called for the bartender. He approached and I remember that he looked amazingly like my Uncle Ron. "Excuse me, sir. I was sitting at that table with my friends. The waitress told me there was some problem with our getting a drink." I said, pointing to my table, Harry, and Tom. "What is the problem? Do you need to see our cards?"

"I'm sorry but I can't serve you" he said, not really looking at my eyes. He started to move away and I said, "Wait, what do you mean, you can't serve us. We're all over 21, we're able to pay." He said, "Look, I just can't serve you, why don't you try the bar around the corner."

Now I'm a fairly easy going guy, one who doesn't look for trouble, but this bartender and his attitude were bothering me. "Look, buddy," I said half sarcastically, "you got to give me more than that. We're here, we're legal, we've got money, and you're open. Why can't you serve us a drink?"

He sighed, rolled his eyes and said, "I can't serve them," motioning to Harry and Tom. "Them," I said, louder than my normal tone. "What's wrong with them?" As I think back now, the innocence of that remark brings a smile.

He said, "Look, buddy, I don't want no problems here. I can't serve them. What if something happens to them? I can't be responsible."

"Happens to them?" I bellowed, "What if something happens to you?" I said, half threat, half truth. "There is nothing wrong with those guys. They are citizens, with money, in a public establishment, and they are lucid — certainly more lucid than you." My defiance was soaring.

"Look, fella," he was now meeting my defiance on equal footing, "I've been a bartender for more years than you've been alive, and I know what I can and don't have to do and I don't have to serve no cripples."

My anger kicked up ten more decibels. "What the hell're you saying. That you refuse us service because my friends have disabilities. Do you know that this is America — that we're in the 80s."

"Look," he interrupted, "You better get out of here before I have to call the cops." "The cops, good, the cops, call them. Maybe they'll remind you that we're in America." I yelled with a point of my finger.

By now I was ready for battle. Like any good street fighter, I looked around the bar for allies. "What do you think about this shit," I said to the fellow to my left. "This bartender said he won't serve me and my buddies because they use wheelchairs." He wasn't interested, didn't want to get involved. I looked to the other side and saw an older, African-American and appealed to him. "How about this. This guy won't serve us cause he has something against people with disabilities." I took a little editorial prerogative, but hey, that's what street fighting is all about. The fella shrugged his shoulder. I tried again. "You would think we were in Selma in the 60s?" He didn't bite and I knew this would be tough.

By this time, the bartender had phoned the police and was again asking us to leave. I said, "No, no way. You'll have to throw us out." I moved from the bar and started to work the crowd. "Can you believe this? Is this really happening in America?" Somehow, I felt the America tie-in might appeal to others in the bar.

I went back to the table to regroup with Harry and Tom. Harry talked first. "Listen Al, let's not cause a scene. These folks don't want us here. We can find another place." "Harry," I exclaimed, "Don't you understand, we don't have to stand for this type of discrimination?" "I know," Harry replied softly, "but what is fighting going to accomplish." Harry is the type of guy who has grown accustomed to the second-class treatment typical for people with disabilities.

Then Tom spoke up. In a labored way, he said, "We're people, too. This is unfair." Tom has always been a fighter, and this incident had his Irish blood boiling.

Soon, the police arrived. Before I could get to them, the bartender ran up and began his story. I approached from the other side of them and introduced myself. The voices raised, and the police asked that we go out into the hall to sort this out. With both sides on the table, the police told the bartender to get back in the lounge, and then turned to me. "Look, Al, we're not sure, but we think this guy does not have to serve you if he feels the drinks may be harmful. It's the same as if a person was intoxicated and was refused service."

"Intoxicated?" I interrupted, "Officer, my friends and I are not intoxicated. All we want is one drink and then to hit the sack. We're not looking for trouble, only the same courtesy anyone else would be afforded."

They were stuck. It was a standoff. Oppression versus justice — a classic American dilemma. They looked at me, then at each other, then back at me as if this problem would just evaporate into the air. Finally, the more kindly of the two said to me, "Al, there is a bar right around the corner. Why don't you get a six-pack and drink in your room?"

I was dumbfounded. It was as if I was dreaming all this up. After a long stare, I asked for their full names for my records, and weakly thanked them for nothing. I went into the bar to fetch my friends, and as we walked out, I couldn't help raise my fist into the air, akin to the black power salute used in the 1968 Olympics by the African-American runners who won the gold and silver medals.

In 1984, I received an intriguing resumé in the mail. It was from a creative man named Tony, who had recently graduated from the University of Pittsburgh, School of Social Work. As an album of that same program, I was drawn to Tony's resumé. More, however, was how he crafted his resumé, different than the ones I typically see. I called Tony in for an interview.

As I was dialing his number, I had a vague recollection that I had heard his name before. As soon as he answered the phone I remembered. Tony had cerebral palsy, and prior to his admittance to the MSW program, I was consulted by the school on his application. That was some four years earlier.

Tony and I set a date by phone, and on the arranged day he arrived early, looking sharp. We sat for a while and made the small talk. I was impressed with his spunk and presence. Soon we were deep into the interview.

I asked a myriad of questions and was impressed with his responses. As we moved toward conclusion, I asked Tony about other places he had applied to for an interview. I had assumed that connecting with United Cerebral Palsy (UCP) was one of his first stops on the interview trail. Then he told me. Ours was his 75th interview. 75! ! !

Now, here in front of me, was a qualified, well-spoken man. He had a University of Pittsburgh MSW. He looked good, he had good placement experiences, and he was obviously intelligent. He was interested in any type of entry-level human services position. He had the Office of Vocational Rehabilitation ready to buy any job aids he needed. And he had been on 75 interviews.

As I paused to appreciate the magnitude of these facts, I caught myself staring at Tony. In a nonchalant way, he asked what was wrong. Was it anything he had said. All I could say was, "You're hired."

Recently, I was pulled into a complex situation. It revolved around the sexual molestation of a child by a person I know. The person accused had a disability, and had exposed himself in front of this youngster, asking that the child strap him with a belt.

As we spent time together, something mandated by the state as preliminary to any court action, his story unraveled. This man had spent his adolescent, formative years in an institution for people with mental retardation. Although I am convinced he is not mentally retarded, his speech and severe physical situation led way to his institutionalization in this particular facility.

During his time in this place, a facility that is respected for its fine work with people with retardation, he was deeply abused by staff. The most flagrant violation he experienced happened when he was prescribed for whirlpool treatment. Given his spasticity, the physiatrist ordered weekly whirlpool baths to relax his tight muscles. During these baths, he would often become so relaxed that he would have a bowel movement in the whirlpool. This caused extra work for the staff. They warned him that this behavior must stop, and when it didn't, they thought he was doing it on purpose. Warnings led way to abuse, and before too long, this man was subjected to an unbelievable punishment. If he had a bowel movement in the whirlpool, the staff member would pull him out of the vat, restrain him on a PT table and them strap him across the buttocks.

This abuse happened regularly over a three-year period. After each beating, he was warned that if he said anything he would be even more severely abused. He said nothing.

All of these situations happened to me or my friends. They happened in Pennsylvania, and they happened in the 80s. There are more, but these three make the point. People with disabilities are devalued and abused in our society today. These experiences are not from another era, in some far-off place, but around us, today.

Further, these situations are all a fallout of devaluation, distantiation, and disempowerment. As far as we have come as a society, we live today with close to 50 million Americans with disabilities subject to abuse, segregation, and blatant discrimination.

1

Disempowered

The God Who Gave us Life
Gave us Liberty at the same Time

T. Jefferson, 1774

1

Disempowered

There are millions of people in the United States who are vulnerable and dependent. Some are children with abusive parents. Others are homeless or people without a viable economic base; still others are frail elderly or those forgotten in neighborhoods. Then there are people with disabilities, some children, some elderly, but most economically dependent and vulnerable to the human service system.

Although specifics on these groups differ, one area in common is disempowerment. For one reason or another, these individuals and groups have limited power. Some lack power because they have no economic base; others because they lost or lack certain skills; still others are distanced from society because they are different. However, all of these groups are stereotyped and stigmatized. They are held accountable to a particular script and treated according to that script.

In most cases, the typical way these groups are treated by government, private organizations, and most citizens, is as recipients of service or goods. That is, an entire service system has developed around people with differences as to create an industry. This industry produces thousands of jobs and organizations of experts keeping the person with a difference as the commodity. These different people then, are devalued in such a way that the system, public and private, sees very little worth in what they can contribute. Consequently, a maze of handouts and services are made available and delivered in such a way that these disempowered groups stay in dependency roles.

Although any one of these groups could be reviewed within the context of interdependence, the focus of attention of this book is on disability and rehabilitation. This chapter explores how people with disabilities become disenfranchised from society and consequently, devalued. This devaluation creates a strong disempowerment, both internally and externally.

Indeed, an entire specialty of human services, known as rehabilitation, has emerged as a system to deal with people who have disabilities. It is prudent for us to explore rehabilitation.

THE GOALS OF REHABILITATION

Whoever undertakes to set himself up as a ridge of truth and knowledge, is shipwrecked by the laughter of the gods.

A. Einstein

Rehabilitation is generally understood to be a process whereby people who have incurred some disability or change to their body function are assisted in learning or relearning these functions (Garrett & Levite, 1973). Having its roots in services to the returning war veterans, rehabilitation has grown to become a viable medical specialty complete with a host of sub-specialties. Today, rehabilitation is a powerful industry unto itself.

The goal of any rehabilitation effort is to first save, then stabilize, and finally restore the individual to the pre-injury state. In fact, rehabilitation is defined as a "holistic process based on comprehensive, ongoing evaluation of each disabled person's specific limitations, abilities and needs." (Goldenson, 1978).

In my experience, rehabilitation efforts boil down to four basic themes. Interestingly enough, these themes are vital to all people. In fact, I feel these four rehabilitation goals are exactly the same as the major life goals of all people.

A SAFE PLACE TO LIVE

All of us want and need a living environment that is safe and secure. We crave our privacy and security and without it feel incredibly vulnerable. Understand here that I am not just referring to a place to live. Although housing is important, my point goes much beyond just environment. Much as a home is greater than a house, a safe and secure environment is well beyond just an environment.

MEANINGFUL THINGS TO DO

We are all multidimensional creatures with a variety of facets to our lives. One important area is found in our daytime activities. For most adults this means a job or vocational part of our lives. In fact, for many of us, much of our identity is wrapped up in our work. When we first meet new people we quickly get to occupational roles. Indeed, status and importance are often linked to occupations. Consider two smartly dressed men who are introduced at a party. Both look good and successful, but once the occupational introductions are made, one is found to be a stockbroker, the other a stock boy. Immediately the caste is set.

People are searching for meaning in their lives. Often, if they do not find it in their occupations, it can be found in volunteer or community work, recreation, or through family activities. However, an important point to consider is that people need to dictate and determine what is meaningful. Yet, these determinations are influenced by the thoughts and wishes of others. This struggle between self and influence of others will be examined further in this text.

INTIMACY

Closeness and relationships breed life. Without intimacy in our lives, the void can be unbearable. Indeed, reports and studies continue to show that without intimacy people fail to thrive. To this extent, developing, keeping, or maintaining intimate relationships is a critical element of rehabilitation. Consequently, as we will cover later in this work, relationships are the most critical dimension of interdependence.

REJUVENATION

The final major aspect I see in rehabilitation, and in fact, to a solid healthy life for all of us, is recreation and rejuvenation. No one can work all the time. None of us can hold up being under the spotlight all the time. To this extent, we must have time and opportunity to refresh and recollect ourselves. If you pause to examine the word recreation, you find the blend of two powerful themes, "re," which means to go back and "create," meaning to start anew. Rehabilitation is about recreation of a lifestyle and any thoughtful approach would dare not forget it.

*Given an ounce of
information, we
make generalizations
as large as a tub.*

G. Allport

REHABILITATION OUTCOMES

When one thinks of these four dimensions from the focus of disability, two major issues jump out. One is that these four themes are important goals shared by all individuals. All of us want, need, and strive to achieve these four goals. Indeed, life doesn't seem to be complete without them. This pushes a powerful point of similarity of being. Yet people with disabilities are often seen as being dissimilar, or different from other people.

The second point is that the rehabilitation discipline has not achieved desirable outcomes in these four areas, for people with disabilities. The literature is riddled with study after study, showing the continued difficulties in housing, jobs, relationships, and recreation opportunities. Further, those positive outcomes that occur, usually stem from segregated approaches that are not the real wishes of people with disabilities. The reasons for this are many and varied and everyone has their theory. However, I believe that the failure and disparity of outcomes are tied directly to our present service approach. By service approach, I mean the infrastructure, philosophy, and design of current rehabilitation efforts. I will refer to service approach with the term *paradigm* and will describe this concept more vigorously in Chapter 2. For now, though, let's again examine the four goals of rehabilitation and look more closely at outcomes.

WHAT USUALLY HAPPENS TO THE FOUR GOALS

SAFE AND SECURE ENVIRONMENT?

There is no question that in a review of housing outcomes after rehabilitation, most people with disabilities initially retreat home with their parents or spouse. Although this seems to be a natural goal, and for many it is, it may not be the best situation for all. In a review of some 40 people in the greater Buffalo area, (Condeluci & Swales, 1990), all experiencing a disability as a result of traumatic head injuries, 32 (85%) were living at home with parents or spouse. However, these people reported that they were not happy being with their parents or parental-like spouse. Similarly, other studies of people with disabilities who live at home reported equal concerns with satisfaction.

For those people wanting to be on their own after an injury, the housing picture is equally bad. Accessible, affordable, and safe housing is virtually nonexistent for people with disabilities. In fact, as the housing market continues to shift and rents rise, more and more people are being forced to consider less and less desirable settings and locations. Most affordable housing is in undesirable neighborhoods or senior citizen complexes. Often, even these options are not physically accessible.

Finally, for those who cannot go home, or need assistance to live on their own, the picture is worse. Very few community programs exist that can offer appropriate supports. Consequently, most people who fit this profile are ultimately institutionalized. In our small Buffalo sample, we found five such people (15% of the total). National research on this phenomena continues to find similar data. Far too many people who need minimal assistance are often totally institutionalized.

In some regards, this trend can be understood, though certainly not accepted. The core of our federal Medicaid system, the one used to underwrite residential supports by most poor Americans, is driven from an institutional perspective. That is, although the residential services needed by most people with disabilities can be paid with government funds, the services are often only available if the person is admitted to a nursing home or intermediate care facility (ICF). Thus, a person who just needs attendant supports can only obtain this service if they are institutionalized. This issue is at the core of medicaid reform which is still being debated in the U.S. Congress.

Even for groups of people who have access to funding through some diagnostic link (such as people with mental retardation labels), most available housing options are group homes, congregate settings, or institutionally oriented apartments. The bottom line here is that even though some of these group homes are on "main street," they are usually run like institutions. In many regards, the deinstitutionalization that created group homes was nothing more than a process of trans-institutionalization.

Recently, I was meeting with some county human service officials to appeal the growing medical thrust imposed upon residents' UCP supports who have mental retardation labels and were previously in institutions. I was pleading that these folks have the lion's share of their free time filled up by a never-ending stream of medical appointments and therapy sessions, all deemed important by the outside case manager who oversees the program. I suggested that we consider a more balanced approach. After all, we were invading their home. After an intense stare, the lead county official said to me, "Oh, but you're wrong. It is not their home — it is a program."

MEANINGFUL DAY ACTIVITIES?

In the area of employment and day activities for people with disabilities the data is equally tragic. Without question, the inequities and discrimination are staggering. A 1986 Harris Poll exploring disability issues found that an unbelievable 86% of people with disabilities are either unemployed or seriously underemployed. Two-and-one-half as many people with disabilities are at the poverty level than any other group. Men with disabilities who do similar work make $2,600 per year less than their non-disabled peers. Worse, working women with disabilities earn some $3,600 per year less than their peers. This puts women with disabilities at the lowest economic scale for workers. All of this, by the way, says nothing about meaningful work, nor does it speak to the countless thousands of people with cognitive and physical disabilities who find themselves in depressing day activity and work/life skill programs.

The story about my friend who had gone on 75 interviews, is the rule, not the exception. Once hired, most employees with disabilities have to work harder than their non-disabled peers. They know that if they slip even a little, they run a greater risk of being fired or disciplined.

For those younger school age individuals with disabilities this area of meaningful day activities is also problematic. In spite of legal initiatives of PL 94-142, the Right to Education for Children with Disabilities, the number of children being educated in separate, and often poorer settings is staggering. In these situations, standards, resources, and activities are usually lower than that of non-disabled peers.

In 1988, I was asked, by the Secretary of Education in Pennsylvania, to sit on a statewide committee to explore the barriers to educational integration for students with disabilities. Although this is not an area of specialization for me, the experience it provided was profound. Indeed, the lessons I learned took me aback.

❖   I found that a large number of children in Pennsylvania, upwards to 14,000 in one county alone, were educated in segregated settings.

❖   I found that Pennsylvania, the birthplace of "right to education" in 1972, had one of the most segregated educational systems in the country.

❖   I learned that the strongest opponents to integrated education are special education teachers and the union that represents them.

What seemed clear in the experience was that the intermediate unit system of special schools was, and is, a powerful entity. In Pennsylvania, we know that separate is never equal, that integration can and does work, that children with disabilities do better in integrated settings and that there is less social stigmatization of students. Yet, separation is a way of life for education in Pennsylvania, and in other states as well.

INTIMACY?

We know that the divorce rate in western society is high. Some estimates put it at the 50th percentile. Allowing for this, the divorce rate for couples where one spouse is injured is even higher. Perhaps more devastating, is that along with these marital break-ups, friendship, and support networks also fade away after injury. Personal testimonies from around the country continue to reinforce the loneliness and isolation felt by people with disabilities. For those who are injured there are tales of abandonment. For those with congenital disabilities it means limited opportunities to make friends.

This is not to imply that all people with disabilities experience loneliness. Indeed, all people are susceptible to times of isolation. It is reasonable to assume that when your outlets to relationships or opportunity to culture friendships are lessened or cut off, loneliness can be heightened.

This area of intimacy, friendships, and relationships is a central theme in the concept of interdependence. Time and time again we see social programs developed for disenfranchised people such as those with disabilities, yet the loneliness and isolation abound. If we just stop to think of the fundamental importance of relationships to everything we do it is not hard to understand why relationships are crucial. What is difficult to understand is why our rehabilitation programs have not sorted this out as critical, or done something about it.

REJUVENATION?

In 1980, a survey was done of people with disabilities in Pittsburgh regarding the areas of service or programs that were essential to them. Needless to say, the laundry list of vital services was listed on the survey poll. They included housing, transportation, jobs, accessibility, attitudes, and the like. Prior to this survey, some of us took lots on which areas would be tops. I was certain that housing, jobs, or transportation would be first on the list. Top on the list, however, was recreation. Certainly, the others were important, but recreation far outpolled its closest competitor, housing.

Without question, recreation is a vital need of all people. Our 1980 survey was testimony to two important facts. One was that recreation was most important, and two, there were precious few recreational opportunities for people with disabilities, in our area. Today, we are seeing more recreational opportunities, but these efforts are often segregated, isolated, or terribly childlike. Arenas, stadiums, and concert halls are all thinking more about people with disabilities who might attend their functions, but are assuming they all want to sit together, as special handicapped sections are the norm...Or places like the YMCA/YWCA are setting up special handicapped swim nights. Similarly, we are finding that groups such as the Shriners, send circus tickets to specialty agencies like United Cerebral Palsy, assuming all people with cerebral palsy must like the circus. Of course, when these "special people" get to the circus, all must sit together in separate handicapped sections. Hardly the typical way people recreate.

All these are examples of how problematic these situations remain in rehabilitation. Yes, we have more opportunity, but the quality and potential to meet new people and to establish relationships and intimacies in these examples (except with other people with disabilities) is poor.

Indeed, I feel frustrated as to why rehabilitation has not done better in these four important areas. We have invested more money, time, and technology in this field than ever before, yet outcomes remain dismal. I am certain rehabilitation planners and professionals care. However, I am not certain, if they think about the way in which they care and more importantly, if their caring has any effect.

The most important thing that we face in the 21st century is a rediscovery of community.

W. Gaylin

The Importance of Community in Rehabilitation

Most people who know, have experienced, or work in the field of rehabilitation would agree that the most important outcome in service to people with disabilities is their return to the community. This is the ultimate measure of success. Interesting enough, the route to this goal, as practiced by most rehabilitation in North America, is by identifying, labeling, fixing, and changing the person's disability-related deficits. This ingrained methodology is seemingly beyond question. It is simply the way rehabilitation works.

Yet, in many regards, rehabilitation is not working. People are not being fully integrated into community. Clearly most energy, focus, or attention in rehabilitation is dominated by the goal of changing or fixing the person with a disability. In fact, in most rehabilitation literature, the concept of community is often an afterthought. That is, experts acknowledge community, but precious few rehabilitation activities really address or incorporate it in their programs. This reflection is culled more from personal observation and experience than literature or research.

Without question, experts in rehabilitation talk about community, but when we examine the outcomes and impressions of people with disabilities, there is often a different story.

One review of rehabilitation literature I did on the "PITCAT" computer at the University of Pittsburgh found that of 288 primary entries that have the word "rehabilitation" in the title, only five also had the word "community," as well. Additionally, the majority of general rehabilitation texts on the market deal primarily with understanding specifics of disability diagnosis or of related medical aspects. Most have a token chapter on community, but clearly it is not key to the text.

This afterthought approach to community is indeed curious if we are to believe returning to the community is the ultimate rehabilitation goal as articulated in rehabilitation definitions. It is even more curious when one considers the poor outcomes and current situation faced by most people with disabilities in society. In many regards, people with disabilities are not satisfied with their community situation.

It is fast becoming known that people with disabilities is the group most discriminated against in America. (Harris Poll, 1986). Study after study reveals that people with disabilities — some 50,000,000 in America - are the poorest-educated, poorest — housed, most unemployed or underemployed. In fact, it wasn't until 1990 that people with disabilities were finally given their civil rights through the passage of the Americans with Disabilities Act (ADA). Without question, being disabled in America leads to incredible limitations and distantiation.

Even with this knowledge and the fact that disability, by incidence, is on the rise, rehabilitation is still practiced in a microscopic and medical way. One interesting manifestation of this trend is found in a review of the growth in the field of head injury rehabilitation.

In 1980, the birth year of the National Head Injury Foundation (NHIF), there were only a handful of programs in America specifically focused on head injury. It should be no surprise to learn that all of these programs were medical, inpatient services. What is surprising is that in 1990 the NHIF Directory of Services reveals that there are over 800 specialty programs, yet less than a quarter of these are community oriented or based. Although there may be some economic incentives in providing acute care, I believe this facility domination is more a testimony to the power and influence of the medical paradigm in rehabilitation.

To understand these trends it is important to look more closely at the concept of deviance how people become devalued and how this devaluation leads to powerful and divisive stigma and disenfranchisement from society. In his book, *In and Out of Retardation*, Burton Blatt (1981) referred to this phenomena as "banishment." He argued that banishment is the most punitive of actions. Yet, formal banishment through institutionalization, or more informal measures like ignoring, offsetting, or clustering, has been the norm for people with disabilities.

Each new reminder of difference strikes the raw spot; deepens the wound.

J.H. Griffin

Deviancy and Devaluation

Deviancy is a term that refers to a difference. Semantically, the word essentially means "different from the norm." In scientific terms something can be positively or negatively different and be referred to as deviant. However, in popular conversation, the term is usually associated with negativity. We might say that a person who is strange or a danger to society is a deviant, even though the word could equally apply to a brilliant scholar or world class athlete.

To appreciate how deviancy relates to disability and human services, it is important to embrace normative analysis. This is a process where any issue can be defined and compared to the general population. In a sheer procedure of counting elements of an issue, a distribution of incidence can be made. This distribution gives a sense of where people fall in comparison to each other *vis à vis* the issue being measured. For example, if we wanted to look at something as basic as height of adult males in your neighborhood, a random poll could be taken and you would record each man's height in your sample. Figure 1 shows the distribution curve of this sample.

Fig. 1

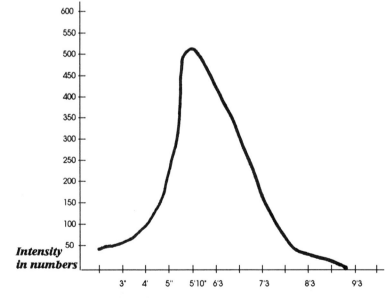

NORMATIVE DISTRIBUTION CURVE

Range in height

As you can see from this curve, the majority of men in this sample are 5 feet 10 inches. This would be called the median height. A man of this height in your neighborhood would fall in the norm. Those much taller and shorter would be on the skewed end of the scale. These men would be deviants from the norm.

If we look at an issue such as physical ability or cognitive skills, again we could do a distribution of function. An interesting difference with this example, however, is found in the context of value. That is, those individuals who fall on the higher level of skill or ability in these two areas would, for the most part, be highly valued. World-class athletes, for example, and any deviance of this group from the norm would probably stand to be rewarded. These rewards may come economically or in a higher profile of status. Equally, the scholar who excels would probably stand to be recognized or acknowledged with awards or citations.

Conversely, the person who scores on the low end of tests or who has a physical situation that compromises their ability to compete, even with the norm, tend to be devalued. This devaluation manifests itself in a number of ways, but all these ways are negative, and in many ways harmful. Indeed, Dr. Wolf Wolfensberger, a leading scholar in looking at devaluation, uses the powerful term, *wounded* to describe the effect of being seen as devalued.

This devaluation is probably most pronounced in two major ways. One is in the actual establishment of fiscal worth of the individual. Daily there are examples of this phenomena in courts across our land. Personal injury claims and trial attorneys have established a legal scheme whereby various functions of people, indeed body parts themselves, are given direct dollar value. In fact, I was once meeting with a personal injury attorney and the issue of worth and physical ability came up in our conversations. I was amazed when he showed me a scale that he uses with clients. This scale literally had a body part and then an ascribed value for that body part. A hand was worth so much, an arm, even more, and so on.

One can appreciate how scales like this have developed. One might even be able to accept some of their usage. When we pause however, in a conscious attempt to understand devaluation, this practice continues to perpetuate the value of those who can, and devalues those who cannot.

The other major manifestation of devaluation is found in the basic structure of our job market. Productivity is emphasized to such a degree that certain skills and abilities make certain people more valuable and worthy than others. This is particularly vivid when we examine lists of occupations and their average net worth.

Again, the economic differential between a doctor and a garbageman seem to be acceptable. After all, we need to have some gauge, yet when these scales or differentials are stripped down to the lowest common denominator, people with cognitive or physical disabilities are usually on the bottom. This devaluation is so powerful that in many cases it has unconsciously affected those who relate to people with disabilities. Most professionals have just accepted the fact that a disability means less economic power and consequently condition their patients or clients to accept less. Story after story is told by people with disabilities about the limited information or encouragement they received, in efforts to pursue dreams.

The Loss of Power and Oppression

Oppression – Overwhelming Control – is Necropholic; it is nourished by love of death, not life.

P. Freire

There has been much written about power — how it is gained and used. These works look long and hard at the topic and give us ideas about how we can be more powerful as people. Few books. However, look specifically at how power is compromised or lost.

In my experience, there seem to be two major routes to the loss of power. One occurs when a person is unable to perform according to some accepted norms in various skill areas. The other is related to individual difference compared again, to certain norms.

Although these two areas can be separate, they are usually tied together in powerful ways. The common bond with both routes relates to the concept of difference and a judgement of acceptable norms. Let's look at both routes separately.

ABILITY

All of us have varying levels of skills in both cognitive and physical areas. The cognitive skills are related to thinking, memory or abstraction of concepts. The physical areas relate to strength, endurance, and dexterity. If we were to create a normative analysis distribution scale and chart where people fall in any of these two major areas or any subset of them, we would find people at various levels of the scale. Of course, there would also be arbitrary parameters of acceptance that would differentiate the acceptable, even at marginal levels, from the unacceptable.

In the general area of ability, the person who falls at the lowest level of acceptance, would be the least powerful. Note, however, that the person at the highest level would still be accepted and probably rewarded. Even though people at the highest level are considered eccentric, they would still maintain their power or have it heightened. This might not hold true in the second major route to power loss, that of difference.

Consider again, the example of the world class athlete, or academic scholar. People at this level are highly valued or esteemed. On the other hand, the person with a disability who cannot move on his own accord, or the person with severe retardation is relatively powerless.

Another key ability factor relates to onset of the situation that led to the ability loss. That is, a person who once had typical, or even extraordinary talent or skill, and then loses it through an accident or illness experiences a power loss, but not nearly as intense of a powerlessness as the person who never had the talent or skill at all. These people (either congenital or childhood emanation) are much more devalued. Either way, a loss or lack of ability in the cognitive or physical areas leads to a loss or lack of power.

DIFFERENCE

Difference is a concept that also relates to the normative analysis scale. However, in this area, I am referring to a difference that is obvious and very deviant from what is considered to be normal or typical.

Recognize that people are creatures of habit with a need to understand their world. We spend countless hours sorting and categorizing things around us. We want things to be predictable and in their place. When we encounter something that goes contrary to our reality, we become uncomfortable. The difference can be color, size, appearance, behavior, age, religion, or any number of factors.

As we look at this concept we must understand that difference has both internal and external impact. On the external side, the drive for order or similarity causes us to set up structure and patterns to our lives. We set up our homes and offices in a way that makes sense to us. If something disrupts or changes our order, we get unnerved. Our rhythms become so ingrained that our habits become mindless. Consider the patterns that you follow each morning getting ready for your day. You probably rise, shower, dress, eat, and then depart your home in very predictable ways. Indeed, when your pattern changes, dysfunction usually occurs.

Internally, we are equally driven for order. This often plays out in the way we attempt to link with people we feel are similar to us. We are social creatures and want to be accepted. In this quest, we work hard to look like, talk like, and act like those we perceive as allied. Conversely, this internal thrust drives us away from those people we feel are dissimilar.

The power of difference is so strong that even if a person has some appearance difference, but is as skillful (or even more skillful) in ability to the norm, will probably be rejected. To this extent difference overshadows ability as a factor in power loss.

This brief review of power loss leads to a more visceral issue — that of oppression. Just that word, oppression can make us uncomfortable. Yet, when you discuss power loss you must introduce the issue of oppression, because people who lose power, become vulnerable to oppression by those who still have it.

Recently, I had the opportunity to attend a workshop on disability and oppression. This gathering, and the substance of information on oppression discussed, was patterned after the Social Issues Training Project conducted by the School of Education at the University of Massachusetts on racism and sexism. Without question, the very roots of oppression faced in issues of race and sex are parallel when we look at oppression and disability.

A person is oppressed when they are held back, either physically or psychologically, from the goals they aspire to, and the norms of society. As stated earlier, oppression is closely linked to devaluation and loss of power.

There are various ways to inspect oppression and disability, but in the University of Massachusetts format, the phenomena starts innocently. Children are born into this world without guilt, blame, or agenda to be oppressive. They then embark on a journey that is influenced by the environment around them. This environment introduces and sanctions oppression.

Now some people will argue that children are not born blameless, but with a natural instinct to oppress for survival reasons. Although each of us have to sort out this innocence/evil question for ourselves, I was drawn recently to a review of this issue in the book, *Life 101*, by John Rogers and Peter McWilliams (1990). As they analyze this question, they come to the simple conclusion — innocent. They justify this conclusion by asking the readers to look into the eyes of babies, any baby . Do we see evil?

In the cycle of oppression, as we age, the sanctioned aspects of devaluation become so omnipresent in our lives, that to oppress becomes second nature. Everyone does it. It seems to be natural. Some people, however, start to question oppression. As they do, the dissonance and pain that follow are powerful. Often it is easier not to question. Indeed, those who question are usually punished. A graphic look at this cycle is displayed in Figure 2. (Harro, 1980).

As we learn more about oppression, we find that there is a scale of actions that relates to behavior (Ploof & Spruill, 1990). This scale (See Figure 3) runs the continuum from active oppression to active interruption of oppression. Subtle or overt, conscious or unconscious, we can all find ourselves on this scale.

Fig. 2.

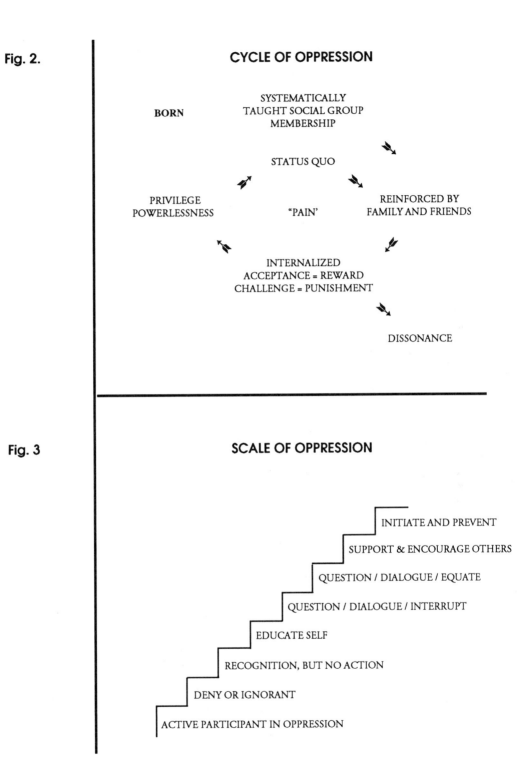

CYCLE OF OPPRESSION

BORN

SYSTEMATICALLY
TAUGHT SOCIAL GROUP
MEMBERSHIP

STATUS QUO

PRIVILEGE
POWERLESSNESS

"PAIN"

REINFORCED BY
FAMILY AND FRIENDS

INTERNALIZED
ACCEPTANCE = REWARD
CHALLENGE = PUNISHMENT

DISSONANCE

Fig. 3

SCALE OF OPPRESSION

INITIATE AND PREVENT

SUPPORT & ENCOURAGE OTHERS

QUESTION / DIALOGUE / EQUATE

QUESTION / DIALOGUE / INTERRUPT

EDUCATE SELF

RECOGNITION, BUT NO ACTION

DENY OR IGNORANT

ACTIVE PARTICIPANT IN OPPRESSION

Make no mistake about it, to interrupt oppression is not an easy task. There are no incentives for it, other than the feeling you get knowing you have done what is right.

Consider this scenario. You are at a party with some old friends. Someone starts a joke that is offensive to some group. What do you do? If you state that you are offended, your friends will probably tease you, or ask how you became so pure. If you press the issue, you are sure to strain your friendships. So most of us just go with the flow. We rationalize to ourselves that we aren't really like these friends; we know better. Yet we still allow the oppression to continue.

As we allow oppression to occur, we set ourselves up for internalized dominance. This concept, articulated by Janet Sawyer and Dorrie Brannock (1990), in their article "Internalized Dominance", explores how the dominant or powerful element of a culture can take hold. The literature, art, and popular products of society allow the oppression to continue. Insidious reinforcement of this power group intensifies.

Given the depth of oppression, its manifestations have taken hold of our culture and institutions. Oppression against people with disabilities is so intense, that our system has adjusted to it. Consider Figure 4, a list of cultural/institutional overtones, articulated in the Oppression and Disability material: (Ploof & Spruill, 1990).

Fig. 4

PLACES OF OPPRESSION	
INSTITUTIONAL	**CULTURAL**
Housing	Values / Norms
Employment	Language
Education	Standards of Behavior
Media	Holidays
Religion	Roles
Health Services	Logic System
Government	Societal Expressions
Legal Services	The Arts
Transportation	
Recreation	

On both columns of this list, reinforced oppression is present. Consider something like logic. In our culture, our logic often takes an either/or perspective. Either you're good or you're bad, strong or weak, capable or incapable. This leaves little room for difference, deviation, or question.

As oppression continues, we see the vexing aspects of prejudice and handicappism flowing into our arts and literature. In a stimulating article, *Handicappism*, Robert Bogdan and Doug Biklin (1975), pointed out the following awareness:

> *Handicappism is a set of assumptions and practices that promote the differential and unequal treatment of people because of apparent or assumed physical, mental or behavioral differences... Ironically, handicappism manifests itself even in the organizations and institutions which have as their official duty the rehabilitation, care, and processing of people who are allegedly handicapped. It seems that most systems that are operating today for the handicapped are based on handicappist principles.... A cornerstone to the handicappism of professional systems is that services to the disabled people are considered a gift or privilege rather than a right.*

The power of oppression and the handicappism that it creates has led to a skewed societal perspective of disability. Indeed, people with disabilities are, in many regards, scripted into preconceived roles. Let's explore these deviance roles.

DEVIANCE ROLES

∞

Social problems stem not from individual deficits, but rather from the failure of the society to meet the needs of all its members.

L. Gutierrez

When we encounter a person who is different, we are cautious, distanced, curious, or hostile. In our efforts to figure out and order the different person, we resort to our past experiences. Some people with disabilities have only recently been visible in society. If we don't understand disability, we will resort to images or ideations that have been developed from books, or things we might have heard or seen in the past. We might conjure up circus sideshow or freak images, or Gothic institutional images. We might think back to a movie image of people with disabilities, or to television portrayals such as telethons.

It is important to realize however that most of these images or past portrayals fit roles of pity, charity, sadness, menace, sickness, or some other less than equal or positive impression. Wolfensberger's (1971) classic work *Normalization* (1971) explores these deviance roles. He shows them as:

Menace

In this situation the person is seen as threat to the community or to themselves.

A strong example of the menace role is found in the community resistance to group residential settings for people considered to be deviant. It is commonplace to find group home proposals being challenged by community leaders through zoning laws. Often these citizens will cite concern for children in the neighborhood if a group home is open. Their concerns are exemplified in positioning the deviant as a menace to the community. It is interesting to note that the Fair Housing Act of 1989 has begun to stop unfair and discriminatory zoning laws that were often used in these cases.

Object of Pity

Pity is often related to a sense of sorrow or of feeling bad for the person. An important point here is that when a person is pitied they can never be respected. Pity and respect are at opposite ends of the same continuum.

As I think about pity, the powerful example of telethons can be used to drive home the point. For the past 30 years, telethons have been used as fund raisers for charitable organizations. Often, telethons are promoted as educational opportunities to help the community understand the ramifications of the deviance. For people with disabilities, this might play out in stories or interviews about them and how they are overcoming tremendous odds.

People knowledgeable about telethons know that it is the pity angle that really sells. As the telethon winds down to its final hours the frenzy of pity crescendos and the pleas and tears begin to flow. In what is now a classic scene, with tie askew, the telethon host is etched in our memories with a beautiful little girl in crutches singing "Mandy." As the camera closes in we can see the tears in the host's eyes as he finishes the song and kisses one of "his kids."

Sickness

Often people with disabilities are automatically associated with sickness or illness. The person is labeled as a patient and must have a treatment plan.

This sickness role is a strong one. Without question, people with disabilities are seen as synonymous with illness. I am often amused by the fact that when a person is discharged from the hospital, apparently recovered from what led to their admission, they are escorted to the door in a wheelchair. I am sure this practice has something to do with liability, but the image of disability and illness is striking. Certainly in most rehabilitation programs, treatment plans designed to eradicate deficits are the norm.

Burden of Charity

The person is seen as being worthless and of little value to society. Only charity is viable for the person.

Charity is often associated with worthlessness. In a charity role, people are perceived as not having much to contribute for themselves, consequently benevolent others must step forward. This charity image is exemplified for me every time I see a friend who I have not been in contact with for years. After initial pleasantries, the topic will always shift to occupations. When I tell my friend that I work for an organization that provides supports to people with disabilities, invariably they will pause, get a warm smile on their face and then tell me how special I am. Then they will tell me how I must be special to work with "them." This example is wrapped in both charity and pity.

Object of Ridicule

In this situation, the person is found to be humorous and the butt of jokes. Often they are made fun of by others around them.

When I think of the ridicule role, I quickly remember a man from my home town who was retarded. This fellow was always pleasant, cordial, and like most of us, hungry to be accepted. As kids, of course, we used to tease Joe-Joe, as he was called. Everyone did.

Then came the day of the ultimate tease. Joe-Joe was delivering papers and, as was his typical course, dropped off a paper at the local tavern. Some men there who had been drinking decided to play a practical joke on Joe-Joe. One man called him to the bar and when he wasn't looking another mixed a glass of beer with some Clorox that was in the corner. They told Joe-Joe that it was a new drink and that he should "shoot it down." Of course, always looking for approval, especially from the men at this bar, Joe-Joe did what he was told. A minute or two after the drink, Joe-Joe collapsed at the bar. He died later that night from a toxic reaction from the drink and medications he used. Sad as this story seems, the real irony was that no one was ever arrested or even challenged for Joe-Joe's death. He was so devalued, that it just didn't matter that he died.

Eternal Child

For many people with disabilities, treatment is from an infantile perspective. Even adults are looked at as if they are children.

The eternal or permanent child role is a deep and in many regards, insulting one. Time and again, I see examples how adults with disabilities are treated as children. As I write these words, I can see out my window my Uncle Pete. A few months ago, Uncle Pete had a stroke. It left him with a left side paralysis and some-word finding (aphasia) problems.

My Uncle Pete is a proud man. He worked hard for his family, raised two great kids, and is a whiz with cars. Now, Uncle Pete is treated, more or less, like a child. At our family outings, people talk down to him and attempt to simplify things to an infantile low. It's not that people want to put Uncle Pete down. Rather, it is this powerful permanent child role that is so closely associated with disability that is the problem.

Holy Innocent

In many cases, the person is positioned as a gift or challenge from God.

This role relationship to deity is a tough one. In my work with United Cerebral Palsy, I have often run into families who associated the birth of a child with cerebral palsy as a challenge or message from God. They were convinced that they were either being tested or punished for some religious reason.

Certainly, peoples' religious beliefs are their own business, but I have a hard time seeing the birth of a child with a disability as some special test. It seems that all of life, for that matter, can be seen as a test. This issue, however, rings a little deeper.

If having a child with cerebral palsy is seen as being more difficult than raising any other child then we need to look, not at God, but at people and society. Why is it harder for a family with a child with a disability? One reason is that people have not understood, nor accepted. Another is because our society has not adjusted to welcome someone who might move, talk, or think differently. These don't seem to be God's problems, but ours.

A few years ago, I had the pleasure of speaking at a conference in New York. I was on the same program as Rabbi Harold Kushner who presented his classic talk on "When Bad Things Happen to Good People." If you know his book by the same title (Kushner, 1979) then you are aware of Kushner's perspective where God fits in a review of bad things. After the birth of his son, who was diagnosed with progeria, Kushner found himself in the horns of a dilemma. As he tried to understand why this bad thing had happened to his family, his first thoughts were that he had done some "wrong" and God was punishing him. Yet in review of his life and actions, he could find no reasons. The next logical conclusion, was that God was bad and uncaring. Of course, he couldn't accept this perspective. So, who was bad? Where did he go wrong? After much thought and prayer he came to the conclusion that neither he nor God was bad, but that at times, in the natural course of life, bad things happen.

Simple conclusion, yet powerful in how it liberates people. Still, the perception that sin and will are related to disability persists.

Thus, this concept of deviance roles is one of vital importance to the interdependence approach. In essence, we have two converging themes, both related to roles. One is the litany of deviant or negative roles that people who are different are cast into. In this regard we have these strong roles that are negative and sanctioned by society thrust upon the person.

The second issue relates to the typical social roles that valued people play. Often, people with disabilities do not have an opportunity to experience or realize these roles. Sometimes, this is because the devalued person has not had the chance, other times it is because the person just cannot perform the role in the typical societal way.

This duality of challenge with social roles gets us to a basic internal/external question that will weave through this work. This challenge is a micro/macro dilemma that needs to be balanced. It is my thesis that we have not adequately addressed these issues. Indeed, I feel that we have focused most of our attention on micro issues of deficits and problems faced by people with disabilities.

In the context of social roles, I see the same emphasis on the micro or internal side. That is, in recent years given the work of people such as Wolfensberger and Goffman, we have a much better articulation of the stereotypic and stigmatic roles that people with disabilities (or any other deviance) are cast into. This has certainly been helpful and important in community work. The concept of interdependence recognizes and embraces these micro issues.

What also needs to happen, however, is to push a balance on macro issues, as well. In this area, we need to look at typical roles and the ways these roles must be adjusted or supported to enable the disenfranchised person to have full access to community.

ROLE EXPECTATION, BEHAVIOR, AND STEREOTYPES

As the goal of rehabilitation is successful return of the person with a disability to the community, the issue of social roles within the family and community is very important. Indeed, a growing number of reviews of reintegration of people with severe disabilities have focused full attention on the issue of social roles (Taylor, Biklen, & Knoll, 1987). A social role is a particular identity that one plays in the course of life (Wolfensberger, 1983).

We all play vital social roles everyday, often without thought or insight, yet these roles are essential to our interdependence and community success. We are men or women, parents, employees, neighbors, citizens, friends, lovers, consumers, volunteers and many more. Through these roles we gain acceptance, friendships, self confidence, skills, knowledge, new awareness, etc.

As we think about roles, there are those that we aspire to through things we consciously set out to do, and those that we are cast into, often without control to adjust or change. For example, we might choose to participate in some volunteer activity to contribute and be seen as a member of the community who gives back. This role might enhance how we are seen by our fellow neighbors.

Conversely, by virtue of our ethnic background, we may be cast into roles associated with ethnic groups that we cannot change. Sometimes we are cast into roles by others that we may or may not want or desire. Just think back to the role you chose or were cast into in high school.

When I think back to my days in high school, I can remember various groups that created roles. We had the jocks who strutted around school wearing their letter sweaters and jackets. Then there were the intellectuals. These folks were the early day nerds with slide rules, glasses at the tips of their noses, and 15 pens stuffed into their shirt pocket. We also had the machine buffs. These guys all had souped-up cars and in fact, looked like mechanics.

As I think of these groups from high school, I recall how some people chose these groups and then fell into the role they portrayed. Others aspired to join various groups, but never quite made it. These folks were usually at the periphery of the group and often teased by the in-crowd. Regardless of the situation, these roles were important to us in identity, friendships, and connections.

Reflection about roles drives home a powerful sociological concept, one that is key to understanding the concept of interdependence; that role expectation leads to role behavior. In this concept, the more one is cast into an expectation that is tied to a certain role, often the power of the expectation alone leads way to behaving within the context of the role. If everyone expects the jock to act a certain way, even in a deviant fashion, usually the behavior follows.

Certainly, the power and effect of role expectation and role behavior can be observed in many situations. Gangs are one group that sociologists have examined in depth for years, (Whyte, 1943). The influence of the gang expectation can push members to do things they know are wrong. Interestingly enough, this role expectation does not have to be negative. Positive actions can be promoted through role expectation, as well.

Along with the promotion of expected behaviors, role identity can produce long and lasting stereotypes. Indeed, my review of the high school jocks, intellectuals, and machine buffs were deep and complete with stereotypic examples of dress, appearance, and behavior, even though it is not everyday that I think about this era in my life. When people select or are cast into certain roles, they are also subjected to the stereotypes that accompany that role.

Classic examples of role stereotypes can be found in looking at ethnic issues. For me, it is my Italian heritage. There are many stereotypes that are associated with Italians. We are thought to be many things. Consider the following perceptions:

❖ To be dark, passionate, and great lovers.

❖ We are strong family people, with long apron strings to mama.

❖ Most often, we're employed in the trades, probably contracting or cement work.

❖ We are religious people with some strange customs, such as the Maloci. This custom, which incorporates oil, water, and prayer, is designed to ward off demons that have been willed upon us.

❖ Most of us are close-knit, but when we fight, we fight. You know, like in the movies, "The Godfather" or "Moonstruck."

❖ And of course, as in "The Godfather," many of us are thought to be associated with Mafia activities.

❖ Our diets consist mostly of pasta and zucchini and we have a weakness for homemade wine.

❖ Finally, we are macho and sensuous people, proudly displaying the gold chain and horn from our necks. It's as if we got issued these pendant at birth, some initial acknowledgment of our ethnicity.

Isn't it interesting how deep and intense these stereotypes are for Italians? Some people reading this may have had little contact with Italians, but probably picked up some of these stereotypic characteristics somewhere along the line. The stereotypes have created a perception, and in most regards, perceptions are reality. Now this is not to suggest that these descriptors are true. Some are, and some are not. The point is, they are known and perceived by some people as a truism.

The obvious conclusion to the point is, if the expectations for some of these characteristics are real to some, they will accept them as such and look for, as well as pick up on, the behaviors that confirm their expectations. People look to affirm that which they expect.

Of course, the other complimentary point is that for some people, if the expectation to behave a certain role-scripted way is present and steady, some role behavior will follow. Thus, you find the person who really does live out the expected role. This self fulfilling prophecy cuts deep (Merton, 1957).

I use the Italian example to highlight the concept of role expectations and stereotypes because it is real to me. You can think of other ethnic groups and roles that are expected that are equally stereotypic. In fact, a number of years ago, long before he became known as America's best loved comic, Bill Cosby made a gutsy educational film titled, *On Prejudice*.

In the film, Cosby is sitting alone, on a stool, in the center of a stage. He is smoking a cigar and his face is colored with white grease paint. As the film begins, Cosby starts to speak out on various ethnic groups. He does not mince words, using powerful slurring descriptors such as nigger, dago, kike, and the like. He reviews the stereotypes of a number of ethnic groups and at first it appears humorous. The tendency for the audiences in training I have shown the film to is to chuckle, because we have come to know Cosby as a funny man. Indeed, we have cast a role expectation for him as a comic. But the slurs go on and go deeper. Usually at this point, my audiences become somewhat uncomfortable, but still put up with it. Finally, the slurs become so biting, usually my groups become turned off.

Perhaps by today's standards, with comedians who attempt humor at any expense, the film, *On Prejudice*, is not as strong, but Cosby did not make the film to get laughs. It is a potent educational film that drives home awareness and sensitivity to role expectations and stereotypes. Further, it illustrates how these stereotypes can have damaging effect.

Role expectations and their effect on stereotyping and behavior have a prominent place in understanding interdependence. As we attempt to reconnect people who have been disenfranchised, we must think about, and strive to understand the nature and effect of this phenomena. We need to discover how much of the role expectations we, as human service workers, family, or friends promote toward people with disabilities. Further, we must think closely about how we promote social changes and needed community services without reinforcing or adding to existing role expectations and stereotypes of people with disabilities.

This point of promoting the role expectation needs to be thoroughly inspected. It is my feeling, that in our zeal to help and bring awareness to the phenomena of disability, we can in fact promote a role stereotype.

This point was underscored when I was recently asked to do a talk to a Head Injury Foundation group on advocacy. When the conference planner called to ask the title and nature of my talk, I told her I planned to discuss how the Head Injury Foundation can make life worse for people with disabilities. The silence at the other end of the line was deafening. "How could you? Don't you know that the Foundation is helping people?" Of course I know that, but I also know that when we push hard to make a point, often we push the most striking stories. Hit them in the gut. This gets attention, but it also perpetuates stereotypes.

We need to remember that the people we attempt to sensitize may become the neighbors of the very people we are supporting to integrate. If they get the wrong message, the results cannot only be confining to those who may share the label and not the stereotype, but long-term in its damage. Initial stories of despair are hard to erase.

Another more subtle promotion of roles is found in our less direct messages, such as logos, names of programs, and brochures. We need to pause here and look at our literature or the material that portrays disability to the public. Although this may seem like a finer point, it is amazing how subliminal and confusing these messages can be. Logos, for example, are the visual portrayal of the program or service. Yet, most human service logos are wrought with pity orientation, or images of deviance or dismemberment. Doves, flowers, and balloons are just a few of the images used to portray or promote people with disabilities in logos.

In his book, *Normalization*, and in the training on "Social Role Valorization," Dr. Wolfensberger takes a close look at human service logos. He reveals image after image of logos and symbols that perpetuate the deviance roles. Disattached heads, pictures of children, clasped hands, sunshine, and the like are standard order for logos.

The National Head Injury Foundation (NHIF) logo is currently under scrutiny by survivors of head injuries who feel it portrays them as childlike and wounded. It shows them as encased in the bosom of their family with a slash through the smallest child's head. They argue that this symbol is not reflective of most people who have survived head injuries. Of course, the people who developed the logo are dumbfounded by this assertion. How could the very people who have relied on the NHIF, take issue with the logo? Others are hurt that these concerns are a sign of rejection by survivors.

The bottom line in this controversy is that the logo does create an image and that image can be misconstrued. Those of us in the circle may know that logo is not meant to harm people. Yet, the logo should not necessarily be for us. In fact, I'd argue that the logo is really for the community, thus we must think about the reactions of the community.

This point is akin to that of labels. Who do labels really serve, and what harm can they do? These are questions that we all need to ask. Today, the label "TBI" is commonly accepted. I even hear people with head injuries refer to themselves as "TBI's." Imagine yourself being known as an initial or a diagnosis. Labels for people dehumanize them.

Program names and other public displays can cut the same way. When parents banned together, years ago to promote an awareness and understanding of retardation, they called them Association for Retarded Children or "ARC." However, over the years, as people with retardation were constantly being treated as children, leaders in the field promoted that the name be broadened. After all, not all people with retardation are children. Soon the acronym ARC was changed to stand for Association of Retarded Citizens.

As services to people with head injuries have proliferated, I am dismayed with the public messages they send. "Heads Up" and "Moving Ahead" are just two titles I have seen to describe groups or other newsletters. Although they may seem cute, they can perpetuate a role stereotype or expectations. These titles call unnecessary attention to the head.

My point in this discussion is not to berate programs and services to particular groups, but to raise our consciousness to the images we can portray. Of course, just as these public items can continue to devalue, so too can the medium be used for positive, image enhancing efforts. Indeed, Madison Avenue knows too well the power of imaging and the message images can promote. Something that is neutral in our perspective, can be juxtaposed with something that is positive, thus creating a spread phenomena to the positive element. A car with a pretty woman. A politician with the flag. In the trade, this is called image juxtaposition, or positioning a product next to a desired image.

Image juxtaposition with things that are negative or devalued are a little more tricky. The concepts can work nonetheless if they are pitched in a way that accentuates the positive.

Consider a recent ad I saw for a cigarette company. Now, we know the dangers of smoking and are reminded daily as to the

risks. To a certain extent cigarette smoking has become devalued. This ad did not let that stop their efforts. It portrayed a
strong looking man with a cigarette. Behind him was the Statue
of Liberty. Superimposed on the ad was a pack of this brand of
cigarettes. The ad said the name of the brand of cigarettes,
followed by "The Proud Smoke." The advertiser has blended the
right amount of positive images with the right words. The net
effect is the strong suggestion that if you smoke this type of
cigarette, you will appear rugged and proud.

The same ploy has been taken with another tobacco company who has developed a national ad campaign promoting the
U.S. Bill of Rights. Although these ads say nothing about their
brand of cigarettes, the fact that the company itself is identified
in the ad is a strong message that they support the rights of
Americans to make choices. The next logical assumption is that
if you are free to choose, you should be free to smoke anywhere
you want.

To a large extent these and other ads create certain expectations about their product. If you buy the car, you'll get the
pretty woman. If you elect the politician, you'll get the allegiance
to the flag. If you buy the cigarettes you'll be proud and free. If
these are things we desire, our behavior will follow and the
advertisers know so.

Thus, role expectation, behavior, and stereotypes continue to
promote a series of devaluation and disempowerment. Although
people with disabilities are caught in the well of oppression,
they are not alone. Indeed, other groups of people who have
become, or have always been devalued, face the same challenges.

As this book focuses on disability issues, it is prudent to
explore past actions and activities designed to achieve rights,
reenter communities or gain power. Most instruction for me has
been to study the civil rights movement, formal change strategies, and the introduction of the independent living movement.
These themes blend and interweave to help our understanding.

LESSONS FROM CIVIL RIGHTS AND FORMAL CHANGE

*I hold it that a little
rebellion now and
then is a good thing;
and as necessary in
the political world as
storms in the
physical.*

T. Jefferson, 1787

As we examine devaluation and disempowerment the lessons
from the civil rights movement are indeed instructive. Major
overviews of civil rights actions articulate time and time again
how precedent and status quo make social change slow and
tedious. (Branch, 1989; Hampton & Fryer, 1990). The dominant
social group in the case of civil rights — whites — continued to
find all types of reasons to resist civil changes. Laws, custom,

tradition, scripture, and history all were used to justify and endorse obvious unfair practices. As African-Americans pushed and resisted, albeit passively, usually levelheaded people did illogical things. Peaceful people became ugly. Quiet people became loud. Religious people embraced sin.

However, perhaps more challenging than these staunch behaviors of the status quo, was the way most southern African-Americans reacted in the early civil rights years when they were approached by those hoping to make changes in the system.

Often, as reformists attempted to organize southern African-Americans to attend citizenship schools or to register to vote, they found these folks not interested. It was not as if these folks liked or enjoyed the way they were treated. Their passivity was more related to the way they were conditioned to accept the second class citizenship status they had held for generations. Quite simply, the years of ingrained discrimination was their reality, as was the preferred status of the whites.

This wholesale acceptance of the status quo is again related to the notion that role expectation leads to role behavior. It is a strong and important phenomena. In the civil rights movement, southern blacks, for generations, were expected to act a certain way. They were strongly expected to be deferential to whites. They were expected to use their own settings and most certainly they were expected not to challenge or question the system. For years and years, the role expectations of compliance and deference led to role behavior of passivity and acceptance. Even logical reasoning and democratic concepts that all men are created equal could not dent these powerful role behaviors.

Another constant question in the civil rights struggle revolves around approach to change. Everyone agrees that things need to change, but how to proceed brings debate. The approach most often associated with early years efforts in civil rights is nonviolent resistance and pressure. Marches, sit-ins, demonstrations, and rallies were all methods where points and press could be made. Later in the movement, some leaders started to advocate more aggressive action. Here the resistance led way to violence on behalf of both sides. Fear became a weapon for change.

This idea of approach can be simplified in looking at some of Saul Alinsky's writings on the matter of change. In *Rules for Radicals*, Alinsky (1969) suggests ours is a world of angles not angels and there are basically two veins to change. One is within the system. The other is outside the system. One is evolutionary, the other is revolutionary. As he builds his case, Alinsky warns of the pros and cons of both approaches.

The evolutionary approach works through the system for change. It is slower, more tedious, and often has compromise built into the results. For the change agent, the results, though somewhat diluted, are often much more stable and permanent.

However, a risk is that the change agent can be coerced in the process. To abate this risk, Alinsky suggests that the organizer must be a political schizoid, capable of working both sides of an issue, and not sell out.

On the revolutionary side, Alinsky tell us that change happens much more rapidly. Additionally, you win more. The risks are that the change is often short term. As soon as your target gets their power base back, they will take back the spoils and often punish the revolutionaries.

Alinsky shows the power basis and change styles in Figure 5. Through this graphic, Alinsky shows that a small number of people at the pinnacle of the pyramid are in power. They are either wealthy, strong, armed, positioned, or in some other way, on the top of the heap.

The middle level is held by those who have some power, but want more. In the course of interdependence, this would be those support people, families, advocates, or friends of the disenfranchised. This class of people are in an interesting position, because they are clearly in the jockey seat between the haves and the have nots. They are positioned to facilitate change, as they have access to the haves. On the other hand, if they are fearful that their assistance to the have nots might compromise their own situation, they are best positioned to buffer them out.

The last level, the have nots, are the disenfranchised. These are the people who have been devalued and, to a large extent, distantiated from society at large. As most of Alinsky's work revolved around economics, he showed the have nots as the largest group of the pyramid. If you consider segments of currently disenfranchised groups, such as people with disabilities, the bottom of the pyramid is not totally accurate. If you consider, however, all groups of disenfranchised people, the numbers swell, and the pyramid analogy gets closer to reality.

Fig. 5

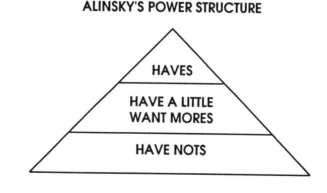

ALINSKY'S POWER STRUCTURE

HAVES

HAVE A LITTLE
WANT MORES

HAVE NOTS

In civil rights, the gamut of actions have been tried. Marches, takeovers, assaults, litigation, legislation, prayers, militancy, riots, elections and on and on, yet we still have serious race-relations issues in this country. It seems as if the nonviolent actions of the 60s coupled with the more hostile actions of the late 60s led way to illusion of change in the 70s. Howard Beach and Bensonhurst are two examples that seem to prove our role problems still exist. It's as if the politics of the 80s have made us comfortable with our bigotries.

This review of civil rights and Alinsky's theory on change is an interesting point at which to examine social actions related to disability. In spite of the depth of oppression, many people with disabilities have begun to speak out. At first, the voices were few and soft. Over the past 20 years, however, these advocates have grown in numbers and passion. Today, we have a viable disability movement, one that is essential to review in understanding interdependence.

DISABILITY MOVEMENT

There must be a beginning of any great matter, but the continuing into the end, until it be thoroughly finished, yields the true glory.

Sir Francis Drake

Although disability has been with society since the beginning of humankind, organized disability activities are commonly recognized as developing in relationship to World Wars I and II. This organization was focused mainly around those who treated or cared for people with disabilities. It wasn't until 1960 that people with disabilities started to question and challenge the system.

In various pockets around the country, courageous people with disabilities began to compare their situation to that of African-Americans in their quest for civil rights. As the civil rights pioneers began to move from the back of the bus, people with disabilities languishing in nursing homes around America began to realize that they couldn't even get on a bus. As the Little Rock 9 pushed for integrated education, people with disabilities and their advocates realized they didn't have access to education at all. Nowhere did the fires of inequity burn stronger about this discrimination than in Berkeley, California. Here a young man named Ed Roberts lay in an iron lung, a prisoner of polio.

At the time, Ed Roberts was a student at the University of California by day, and a nursing home resident by night. He was relegated to a world that treated him as a medical entity. Forget Jim Crow, Ed Roberts had no rights at all. Like most reformists however, Ed had a strong and vivid mind. As he watched the nightly news parade of civil rights activities he realized two important things. One was that civil rights is a concept that should apply to all people, including people with disabilities. More important, however, was that the road to civil rights is found in organization. In this realization a movement was forged.

Ed Roberts lost no time in starting this movement. With colleagues at the University of California he founded the first Disabled Student Services. This organizational energy soon spread and shortly thereafter the first Center for Independent Living (CIL) was founded in Berkeley. (It is important to note that in parallel, yet unrelated activities the development of CILs, as they are known was occurring in Boston and Champaign, Illinois.)

As with the other civil rights movement, the CIL efforts in the late 60s was slow and tedious. Old norms change and adjust slowly and resist every step of the way. Add in the powerful and ingrained stigmas associated with people who have obvious and severe physical disabilities and the concept of equality becomes that much more difficult. Consequently, the movement jelled slowly. Money was hard to come by as government agencies did not trust people with disabilities. Their perspective was that people with disabilities are to be treated and helped, not funded directly. An even more fundamental problem was a name and identity to build from.

Roberts and other national leaders with disabilities went around the horn on the issue of identity. A focused definition to capture the movement's goal was needed, but the format of the movement also needed to be separate from traditional rehabilitation efforts.

In the early 70s, a series of national gatherings were held to cement the movement. These forums consisted of mostly people with disabilities, and although some non-disabled people did participate, all decisions were clearly initiated and ratified by consumers.

Perhaps the strongest issue, one that still is at the core of most debates on interdependence, is the theme of consumer control on choices. Disability leaders felt that people with disabilities must have control of their lives and the programs that are designed to assist them. This led way to a key principal of independent living, that of consumer control of the CIL's. It was ratified that all CIL's must be at least 51% governed and staffed by people with disabilities.

The underlying principle of this dictum is found in the importance of peer relationships. Leaders of the movement felt that those who could most clearly understand an issue are those who have struggled through it. Much like Alcoholics Anonymous, peer relationships in the disability movement are critical to its efficacy.

Another critical point in the movement that occurred in 1975 was the consensus definition of independent living, painfully culled at these national gathering of disability leaders. After a full week of debate and discussion, the following definition was chosen:

Independent living is control over one's life based on choice of acceptable options that minimize reliance or dependence on others.

This definition went on to be adopted by the federal Rehabilitation Services Administration and inserted into the Rehabilitation Act of 1973, as amended in 1978. This was monumental to the disability movement for it was the first time government acknowledged independent living as a viable concept. It also paved the way for federal and state funding for the creation and development of Centers for Independent Living around the country. Ed Roberts' dream in the early 60s was finally realized and more importantly, sanctioned.

Today, the movement struggles with new, but equally challenging issues. If interdependence is to be gleaned from the fruits of the disability movement, it is imperative that we explore and address these issues. Key among the questions of the 90s are:

Service Provision vs. Advocacy

The growth and development of independent living centers and programs initiated with advocacy. Without advocacy, key services, such as attendant care services and peer counseling, would not have occurred as soon. Indeed, advocacy led way to an entire movement. Yet, as advocacy created the movement it also created bureaucracy. Over the past 20 years of the movement, it is interesting to watch the shift. First the outspoken advocates criticized the system and started a movement. As the movement fueled, these same advocates became the persons running the programs. Of course they vowed to do them better in services to people with disabilities. Then the hard questions had to be answered.

How can massive service needs be administered with limited resources? Now all of a sudden, the advocates began to talk like the old bureaucrats. Without question, when you become a service provider, you can lose some of your voice as an advocate. If the CIL's have problems with the way the system makes decisions, and raise concerns, they run the risk of losing their contract, especially if the contract is tied (as most are) to the system making the decisions.

Further, as the CIL's grow and develop around these contracts, infrastructure components such as buildings and common services, get tied into existing contracts. Thus, a lost contract can have devastating effects on the IL Center or program. This insidious linkage can cause deep and often ethical compromise to a system.

A recent situation I had with a CIL illustrates this conundrum. This organization has an attendant service program, and worked hard to pull it off. All through the advocacy phase, the CIL networked with various groups as to the importance and viability of attendant services. However, once funded and faced with some uncomfortable decisions as to who is eligible and who is not, the CIL had to become selective.

I approached them on behalf of an individual who, although associated with one of the disability groups, was not deemed eligible for services. I challenged them on this. It was clearly a different tune from the advocacy period. The CIL responded that I just didn't understand their situation. They only had so much money and could not serve everyone. When I asked if they could advocate or lobby for consideration of people such as my friend, they said they would. They also warned me not to expect too much because the system was doing all that it could. This seemed to be a classic sellout. Prior to the award of their program, they welcomed everyone's help. However, once in the "game," however, they became bureaucratically cautious.

Role of the Non-Disabled

Non-disabled people have always posed a problem in the independent living movement. Initially, they were the reason that services and opportunities were limited. Now, they continue to muddy the waters as they bore their way into the movement from a staff and volunteer perspective. This leads to an interesting debate. Are they friend or foe? Are they helpful or harmful to the movement? Should they be on the inside or outside.

In spite of these situations, the truth of the matter is that non-disabled people are indeed within the movement and the trends are showing that they may be running the movement. In two major states, Pennsylvania and Michigan, non-disabled people seem to rule the roost. Out of 16 programs in Pennsylvania as of July 1990, 12 were being run by people who do not have a disability. In Michigan, non-disability influence is even greater. Seven out of nine programs are guided by non-disabled. If this isn't enough, out of all these programs in both states, 12 out of 15 are volunteer-led at the board level by people who have not experienced a disability.

A further point of confusion in this whole matter is the general question of what constitutes a disability. A disability is thought to be a tangible interference in carrying on basic life tasks. This interference should be physical, cognitive, or emotional. Further, it could be temporary or permanent.

An interesting notion on disability was advanced by Frank Bowe (1978), in his book, *Handicapping America.* He states:

> *The concept that handicaps result from interactions between disabilities and environments is well illustrated in primitive-culture; survival depends upon strength and agility, so physical disabilities become handicapping.*

In this perspective, one is only handicapped when the interaction between the individual and the environment is interrupted. If something can augment the interruption, the handicap would be removed. The disability, however, would still be present.

When I meet people from around the country who are employed by a CIL who do not appear to have a disability, and ask about consumer control and leadership, I often get defensive reactions, or a veiled attempt to justify their involvement and understanding through an experience that left them feeling disabled, such as a break up of a marriage, or a parent's death with cancer. Or the person uses some other justification as to why they should be where they are in the agency.

Now I don't ask these questions to pass judgement or make people feel defensive. It's simply that I am curious about this powerful concept of consumer control and am trying to sort it out myself. What constitutes a disability? Certainly we have the traditional cognitive or physical limitations that affect certain life function areas. Yet today disability is becoming more and more nebulous. Someone who was psychologically abused, or a person who, through economic hardships, has become homeless, might have a legitimate right to claim a disability. So who is or isn't disabled?

Once, during an informal gathering of independent living leaders at a national conference, I was aggressively challenged by a fellow from California who happened to have a disability. We were all sitting in Ed Roberts' room discussing trends and needs and this man questioned me and my right to be there. How could I understand the real elements of the movement?

As a sighted, hearing, walking, talking, and reasonably intelligent person, I represented the very enemy of the movement. Further, since I worked for an agency that addressed independent living issues, I was holding a job that a person with a disability should be holding. Not only was I the enemy, but I was sapping money that should be going to someone within the movement.

Now, I'm not sure how, or even whether this issue is good or bad. If a person is concerned with injustice and oppression, then I believe there is a place for them in the independent living movement, regardless of their physical or cognitive situation. I feel the more who are convinced, converted and become active in the disability movement, the better and quicker the results in addressing oppression. I also feel, however, that people with disabilities must be out in front of this effort. The gains of image, sensitivity, and understanding depend on this positioning and all of us must work hard to make them happen. This issue must be addressed and resolved in the 90s.

Relationship with Traditional Agencies

As the disability movement pushes for some transition of services from traditional rehabilitation agencies to the CIL's, the issue of relationships becomes paramount. No matter how good it sounds, the traditional agencies are always resistant to relinquishing "business" to any one, let alone people who have disabilities. In fact, the drive for most traditional agencies is to get bigger, not smaller. Additionally, many agency directors have intimated to me that they don't think the CIL's could do a better job anyway. This basic distrust is sure to cause problems.

Certainly CIL's are here to stay, but so too are the traditional rehabilitation agencies, at least for now. As we move into the next century, interrelationships between these agencies are a must. Large scale mistrust or warring will only serve to hurt all, and most deeply people with disabilities who need supports.

Need for New Leaders

Related to the previous point on the role of the non-disabled, as independent living programs have grown there has been a void in finding viable leaders. Indeed, this is the number one reason (or excuse) that non-disabled people have been elevated to leadership roles. Regardless, independent living problems have grown so quickly that the pool of available and qualified leaders have not kept up. This situation leads to a serious question of culturing leadership in the 90s.

It seems that actions must be employed that prepare and promote new leadership. One idea, that is directly linked to interdependence, is mentoring. If non-disenfranchised people, especially those associated with specialty rehabilitation organizations, were to identify one or two of their constituents, and brought those people to all of their routine meetings and gatherings, I believe exciting things will happen. One is that disenfranchised people will become better prepared for leadership roles. The second gain is that the mentor himself, will learn, or become re-sensitized to some important lessons about the points of disenfranchisement. Mentoring, a simple process with powerful results, can enhance leadership for the future.

Bureaucratization of IL Issues

One hallmark of the IL movement has been its focus on individualization. People within the Independent Living movement have advocated long and hard against the practice of lumping and stereotyping disability groups. Many human services attempt to box people and their issues. The IL credo, on the other hand, has promoted that people are unique. In this spirit, some people, their goals and needs, don't fit traditional human services. This implies that services must bend for the people who are serviced.

Even with this philosophy and approach, many IL programs are chiseling their clients to fit the human service bureaucracy. This trend and its net effect is frightening to the more idealistic people in the movement. If independent living yields to this bureaucratization, many feel that key strides will be lost.

All of these IL trends for the 90s are important to the concept of interdependence, for it is the independent living movement, more than any other trend, that has advanced the need for a new infrastructure for human services. Indeed, a summary of these points is a prerequisite to understanding interdependence. They are:

- ❖ A balance between providing direct services and advocacy.
- ❖ A balance and clear understanding between the action and roles of people with and without the elements that have created the devaluation.
- ❖ A balance and recognition between the old guard and new approach.
- ❖ An importance in developing and inviting new leaders into the field.
- ❖ A pragmatic realization that even new ideas are subjected to the quick perversions of the bureaucracy.

These trends are all bellwether actions that lead the guard from one dominant theme to a new, emerging theme.

The history of the independent living movement is critical if we are to understand the concept of interdependence. Key points of the struggle all play a part in casting new trends. Indeed, themes from other movements are also part and parcel of the interdependence core. Civil rights and human rights movements have set the stage, but nowhere are these movement themes generically as dominant as in independent living and the disability movement.

Equally important to interdependence is to examine how human services function today and the paradigms that influence these services. Without question, the concepts and themes related to disability have set in motion an active service thrust. For the most part, this thrust has created barriers to the many goals for community integration. To understand and incorporate interdependence, we must understand the nature of services today and the paradigms behind them.

Unreality is the true source of powerlessness.
What we do not understand, we cannot control.

C. Riech

2

Understanding Paradigms

2

Understanding Paradigms

THE PARADIGM

Throughout this work I will be using the term *paradigm*. Although the word usually applies in scientific circles, we can aptly use the term and concept in looking at human services.

A paradigm is the framework in which we look at a problem and answer the questions posed by the problem. It is drawn from the Greek word *paradeigma* which means an example, model or pattern. Most often it refers to the foundation from which the service or action flows. It sets the tone for current and future movement.

In most any enterprise, business, science, education, government, or human services, a paradigm of operation can be found. Although there may be some specific differences, by and large, there are major themes that are identifiable in the larger paradigm that can be ascribed to any of the aforementioned areas.

The term and concept of paradigm was popularized in 1962 by Thomas Kuhn in his book, *The Structure of Scientific Revolution*. In this work, Kuhn investigated the phenomena of shifting paradigms as they related to physics. He discusses how paradigms become dominant and self protective, thus when a scientific discovery pushes thinking toward a new paradigm, strong resistance from the prevailing paradigm occurs. He cites a number of examples of scientists, who, over time, came to challenge existing paradigms and were discredited, disregarded, or shunned. Kuhn suggests that these actions are a result of the protective nature of the prevailing paradigm that is being challenged.

Consider Galileo. In his time, the prevailing astronomical paradigm on the nature of the universe, was that the earth was the center of activity and the sun revolved around the earth. Indeed, the paradigm found this an easy factor to observe. Every morning the sun would come up in the east, move across the sky during the day and then set in the west. How could anyone challenge this notion?

Yet, that is exactly what Galileo did. Using his crude telescope, and charting the stars, he was convinced that the sun was not circling the earth, but that it was the other way around; the earth was revolving around the sun.

When Galileo started to report his observations and ideas, he was not met with support. In fact, his suggestions were so challenging to the prevailing paradigm, and those who had invested in it, that he was seen as a heretic. Even though he attempted to scientifically show the basis for his assertion, he was still ignored. Quite simply, the paradigmatic shift was just too radical, even for the logical, thinking scientists of the day.

Although Kuhn's discussion of paradigms revolved around the physical sciences, the concept of paradigms is relevant in human services as well. One interesting example of a prevailing paradigm that is currently under attack, is education, where, as the shifting occurs, the battle lines are being drawn.

The prevailing paradigm for structured western education is found in what has been called the banking approach of education. This approach is characterized by its narrative and memorization thrust. That is, at its core, the banking approach mandates that the teacher narrates and the student listens. In this process the student stores or "banks" information for future use.

Although some may argue that this is too simplistic an education notion, remember, this narration character is at the core of the banking approach. Teacher talks, student listens and remembers. Everyone reading this book has grown up with this basic notion of education.

I remember in school, how I couldn't wait until I became a teacher so I could talk, and others could listen. I was indoctrinated well into the banking approach of education. So were you! The more we memorized, the further we could go. It often didn't matter if we even understood the material. What mattered was that it could be recalled. The educational paradigm is detailed later in this section.

In understanding paradigms, it is important to note that prevailing paradigms are not threatened until new approaches are found to be successful. Kuhn called these new approaches anomalies. These are actions with roots outside the existing paradigm that are found to work. Most often, these anomalies are approaches developed by entrepreneurs and targeted to the most difficult of paradigmatic challenges. As these anomalies are found to be successful, they begin to threaten the existing paradigm.

In Kuhn's perspective, the approach taken in the anomaly begins to push the prevailing paradigm to adjust or shift. Indeed Galileo, and his charts and graphs of the stars were an anomaly in his time. In their accuracy they began to shift the prevailing paradigm of how scientists saw the state of the universe.

Note, however, that anomalies are not welcomed by the paradigm. Although they offer successful approaches to the problems of the paradigm, they create a much greater threat, the security of those who are embedded in the status quo. Consequently, the existing paradigm promotes that all new advances stay anchored to the paradigm. In many examples, new approaches are even discredited, sabotaged, or destroyed.

Consider typical scientific research found in the halls of academia. Doctoral students are pushed to develop and test new assumptions, but are held accountable to anchor their assumptions to existing literature. Rather than challenge paradigms, the emphasis on doctoral research is on entrenching the existing paradigm. Often it is not until well after doctoral work that we find real breakthrough research.

The notion of paradigms was further explored by Joel Barker (1985), in his book, *Discovering the Future: The Business of Paradigms,*. As his title implies, Barker's thesis applies paradigm shifting to business opportunities. His analysis, none the less, is applicable to human services as well.

In his book, Barker defines a paradigm as "a set of rules and regulations that:

- ❖ defines boundaries; and
- ❖ tells you what to do to be successful within those boundaries."

His analysis is helpful as he describes how old paradigms start to be challenged by what he calls "paradigm shifters." He contends, these people will produce anomalies that challenge the existing paradigm because they are either naive, an outsider to the old paradigm, or an insider who likes to tinker.

Barker suggests, that although the tendency is to reject the anomaly, there are always some who embrace the findings of the "paradigm shifter" and start to apply their approach. These people he calls "paradigm pioneers." As the anomaly begins to create a new paradigm, it picks up steam, more and more "pioneers" join the fold. In Barker's analysis, paradigm pioneers can be in a good business position to take advantage of new marketing trends. Further, these paradigm pioneers lend the energy to create a shift from the status quo, to a new paradigm.

More recently, the concept of paradigms has been applied to aspects of personal change. In his hugely successful work, *The 7 Habits of Highly Effective People*, Stephen Covey (1989), relates paradigms and paradigm shifting for personal consumption. He suggests that paradigms are the way we see the world. They focus our perceptions, understanding, and interpretation of the world around us. To Convey, it is easiest to understand paradigms as a sort of map of the territory; a theory, explanation or model.

In human services, I believe the analysis of paradigms apply as well. In the 30s and 40s new ideas in human and civil rights were advanced. The paradigm shifters of this era were people such as Reinhold Niebuhr, Myles Horton, Saul Alinsky and others. These shifters gave way to pioneers such as Martin Luther King, Jr., Ed Roberts, Burton Blatt, and others.

Indeed, it is interesting to me that a number of key books influential in understanding interdependence were published in the 70s. Books were produced by both paradigm shifters and pioneers. Some that advanced an Interdependent mind set were:

❖ *Rules for Radicals* - Saul Alinsky (1969)
❖ *Asylums* - Erving Goffman (1961)
❖ *Creation of Settings* - Seymore Sarason (1972)
❖ *Normalization* - Wolf Wolfensberger (1971)
❖ *Medical Nemesis* - Ivan Illich (1976)

Looking at human service today, I think we are well into the midst of a paradigm shift. More and more we are finding clients of services dissatisfied, or more importantly, not appropriately served by our prevailing paradigms. Welfare recipients are often angry at their caseworkers; veterans have little good to say about the VA; people with disabilities are dissatisfied with sheltered workshops and on and on.

Why this dissatisfaction? Why are the very people who services are designed for, unhappy with these same services? These questions can only be addressed after an examination of the nature of our services structure as it exists today.

Human Services Today

It is interesting to note that organized human service is a rather new phenomena. Services specific to disability have only originated since World War II, however, it is not my intent here to do a focused overview of the development of human services. There are much more in-depth and scholarly works available on this subject than I can produce. What I would rather do is examine the formation and structure of existing services.

It is my contention that if the current system is not producing the goals people want, then we must examine the structure of these programs. Perhaps the reason the job has just not been done is system failure.

In looking at human services, I have been guided by an exceptional book, *The Creation of Settings and the Future Societies*, by Seymore Sarason (1972). In his work, Sarason suggests that a setting is created when two or more people get together in new or sustained relationships to attain agreed upon goals. It can be as basic as a man and women coming together to create a home and family, or as complex as a band of men and women coming together to overthrow a government.

For the purposes of my overview of human services today, we can apply Sarason's analysis. Most services for disenfranchised people are settings created for an expressed objective. For people with disabilities, these settings might be skill building services, vocational services, residential settings, or other like programs. In any case, these settings are forged from a pre-history that relates to experiences, paradigms, and intent. Sarason offers four factors that are critical to the creation of a setting. These are motivation, values, personality, and power. Each of these factors blend to forge an identity and energy to the setting.

Beyond Saranson's points, I feel other important issues must be addressed as we look at human services today. These form around the setting recipient and setting intention. For this review, these factors will be addressed, exploring seven features of human services today. These are:

- ❖ Focus
- ❖ Leadership
- ❖ Services
- ❖ Space
- ❖ Vision
- ❖ Staff
- ❖ Planning

FOCUS

Most services for people with disabilities have emerged from a focus of seeing the client as having problems that need to be fixed. In this effort to fix people, the system has developed articulate methods to measure deficits and has fine tuned skills and specialities for this purpose.

For the most part, specialization of services has fallen into two major categories; topical or diagnostic. By topical, I mean that some services are specialized in a topical area such as housing, counseling, family issues, recreation, transportation, skills training, employment, and the like. In these topical areas, the organization has emerged as an expert in understanding the topic and is recognized in the community for applying the topical specialty to people with disabilities.

The other major area, diagnostic, implies that the organization has a speciality in some particular disability type. Examples of diagnostic organizations would be those specializing in cerebral palsy, head injury, mental retardation, autism, homelessness, epilepsy, and the like. Indeed, there seems to be no malady that has gone unorganized.

Topical or diagnostic, it is important to note that the focus of most human service organizations is microscopic and oriented toward some speciality. Either group would probably state that the primary intent of their existence is to serve a particular disability clientele; that they are there for the "disabled." This created a paradigmatic climate that continues to promote and verify the importance of the specialty. That is, although the intent of the setting is to liberate the client in a particular specialty area, they can, at times, perpetuate the problems of their specialty.

To this issue Sarason states:

> *To the extent that a setting becomes more and more focused on its relationship to the outside world, it increasingly loses sight of what it can or must do for its own members. This development is inevitable in those instances where the settings are conceived and justified only in terms of what it does to others.*

This focus tends to overemphasize the deficits faced by the recipients of service in the topical or diagnostic areas. Often intense pressure to specialize and the emphasis on deficits pushes the organization to find even more problems that can be solved by the specialty system. To this extent, the system breeds more problems for its specialists to solve. Indeed, if the problems were to all be solved, what would become of the system? Although this sounds cynical, in an unconscious way this can (and does) happen.

A good example here would be the March of Dimes. This group developed out of an objective to cure polio. Once the Salk Vaccine was produced to achieve this objective, the March of Dimes broadened their agenda to address all "birth deficits." Other examples of this trend are found when an agency creates a new service to address further "needs" of their constituents. My own organization, UCP of Pittsburgh, recently did this. For years we have offered independent living skills training. As recipients of this service have attained skills and moved into apartments in the community, we extended our service to incorporate supported employment. These kinds of actions are typical for human services today.

Sarason also reminds us that at times the setting could become fixated on those providing the service and the objectives insidiously shift from clients to staff. That is, the organization and its predominant focus ends up to promote and support staff, over and above the recipients of services or the public at large. In this spirit, it is important to sort out who is really benefiting from the setting or service.

In my experience, I have visited many organizations that report to be client-centered, yet most of the organizational structure revolves around convenience for the staff. Times that services are rendered, where they take place, and how they unfold are often scripted for the staff.

VISION

The vision of an organization is tied heavily to its focus and the paradigm behind its approach.

If the organization has a strong propensity to specialize, its vision would revolve around research and continued inquiry into the elements of the problem. To this extent, the organization gets caught up in finer and finer elements of looking at the problem. For many organizations, who see their clients as the ones with the problem, this means detailed analysis of the person with the disability. An example of this might be an organization with a diagnostic specialty in head injury. Their vision to know more about head injury pushes them to do a more detailed differentiation of people with head injuries. As they do this, they may now divide their clientele up into groups of people with frontal lobe damage, another group with primary temporal lobe damage and the like.

Another manifestation of vision might find the organization driven to find new and safe environments for those individuals who just cannot be fixed. Here, a mixture of specialization and inward vision forge to produce a new product for the hard-to-fix person. In many instances, this concern for protection has resulted in a variety of "settings" for vulnerable people that are isolated and excluded from the community at large. Today, in services to people with head injuries and those with mental retardation, you can find ranches, farms, mountain top retreats, and isolated group homes.

Although they seem to be strongly related, a key difference between vision and focus is that vision relates to tomorrow and focus revolves around today. Vision promotes a future state, but as Sarason so aptly reminds us, future states are tied heavily to the present and pre-history, and this relates to focus.

LEADERSHIP

Typical human services leadership consists of either a president, chief executive officer (CEO), or director. The leader is administratively and programmatically responsible for organizational actions and decisions. Although styles may vary in participation or input from staff, the final say is usually that of the leader.

For the most part, these leaders have gained experience in the particular focus and specialty of the organization. They probably have some formal educational background that has prepared them in the focus or specialization. Usually, they are heavily invested in the paradigm and vision of the organization.

Another safe assumption is that the leader probably does not have the condition (for the diagnostic organization) or difficulty in the topic (for the topical organization) that consumers of service have. That is, if the organization has a specialty in housing, it would be safe to assume that the leader does not have housing problems presently in his life. This is not to say that he may not have struggled in this area, or can't appreciate how homeless people might be feeling. None the less, the leader is usually not a peer to those who receive services.

A final aspect of leadership is found with the board of directors or advisory council. This forum is comprised of enlightened volunteers who are engaged and committed to the focus and vision of the organization. They often, however, perceive their role out of a charity perspective and "donate" their time. In other cases, the leaders of these boards or councils are professionals in rehabilitation themselves. Again, this is not to suggest a negativity in their concern or action. It is more a reminder of how tight and inward many human services can be toward their paradigm. Further it suggests a predictability of leadership in promoting and defining the focus and paradigm. It might also help us to understand why human service organizations continue to blame their clients for continued poor outcomes.

STAFF

Most human service organizations today are staff specific, with the bulk of their budgets going to salaries. Additionally, as charities for people who are societally devalued, monies are often limited and hard to come by. This under-budget phenomena often leads to inexperienced and underpaid staff. Further, for most organizations, the table of organizations for services puts the lowest paid (and usually the least experienced) closest to the consumers of services. This point alone is an interesting one related to Sarason's question of intent. If the consumers of services are most important to the organization, isn't it curious that the lowest paid and least experienced would be in positions closest to them?

Regardless, the manifestation of this trend is that the service is usually tentative and often of limited quality. Even with great supervision, when you mix inexperience with complex situations, the results are sure to be speculative. Again, I must underscore that the staff and supervisors are not bad people who want to do anyone a disservice. It is more to the point that the focus and paradigm behind the focus are so traditional and time worn that people hardly think to question them.

SPACE

Another interesting point when looking at human services today is to examine physical elements of the settings. This can be done by looking at where staff spend their time compared to where consumers of service spend theirs. Although they are far from luxurious, staff quarters are probably apart from and somewhat nicer than the space used by consumers. The separateness is clearly etched when looking at personal space such as bathrooms or lunch areas. In most settings, I have toured, staff have separate quarters on both counts and you can be sure that the consumers know the difference, even if they are not marked or labeled.

Wolfensberger (1971) did an interesting analysis of the use of buildings and space in human service settings. He suggests that buildings can be created or adapted for the convenience of a number of different people or groups; the architect, community, staff or client-user. In looking at the convenience of staff he states:

> ❖ Many buildings, when entered, leave little doubt that the staff convenience was paramount in the designer's mind. Characteristic elements may include segregated staff lounges to which care-

takers withdraw for meals, coffee, rest, etc. and air-conditioning for staff, but not for clients.

❖ Caretaker stations which provide maximal visual control over client user areas, while minimizing staff involvement; the glass enclosed nursing station is a classical example.

❖ Services such as classrooms, beauty shops, barber shops, and therapy areas that are located inside the residential buildings, saving staff the effort of dressing residents, escorting them to other buildings, or arranging for them to leave the grounds.

Aside from these aspects of convenience, the building can also be use to control the consumers and their actions. These settings can give off some powerful images about the nature of the person who uses the building.

I remember my first experience with this phenomena. As an undergraduate, I wanted to do a paper on retardation. Having a close first cousin with this label, I was interested in learning more so I called our local Association for Retarded Citizens. They suggested that I visit a nearby facility to get a better picture. As I drove the initial 30 miles outside the city I was curious about why the facility was so far out in the country. As I entered the grounds, I drove through a large gate, and although unguarded, it offered an imposing first impression. At the main building, I told the outside guard I was there to see the social worker. After being paged by the inside guard, she met me at the main building and we chatted for a few minutes. Then, we were off to "see" the residents. We drove to a large, windowless building about two miles from the main building. As we walked up to the building, she rooted through her purse and pulled out the largest key ring I had ever seen. Fumbling through the barrage of keys, she unlocked the first door. This entry led to an alcove where she fumbled again for the right key to the second locked door. Of course by now, my mind was racing. I was 30 miles from town, through two sets of guards, through two sets of locked doors in a large windowless building. What could possibly lie ahead?

As we entered a large gym-like room (no basketball hoops or sports equipment though), a group of people were huddled at a corner of the room around what appeared to be a teacher. Upon hearing the door slam closed, they turned and stared at us. Next, they all got up and ran, some walked, other scuffled, to where we were standing. I had never before seen so many odd-looking people. Sure, I have a cousin with retardation, but she lives in the community and does the same things we all do. This was clearly, and powerfully different.

This story is vivid for me for a number of reasons, but I share it here as a strong example of not just how settings can control, but the marked image they present. These people were contained and controlled. Everything I experienced that day reminded me, and them, of this fact.

In looking at human services today, we need to consider more than just the settings. We need to examine and review the message of the settings. What does it say about the intent of the services? More importantly, however, what does it say about the people who receive the services?

SERVICES

Although specifics of direct services will differ from program to program, depending on the topical or diagnostic focus, most human services for people with disabilities will look similar. In fact, if one were to visit a different city and seek out the human service organizations (as I often do as a consultant), you would probably find a familiar picture. That is, one would usually find humble settings in the commercial area of the city. The building would be the center of activity, with consumers being bused in and out. Probably the staff would have offices in the same building but offset from where the consumers are located. These offices would be small, cluttered and adorned with posters and sayings on the walls that are inspirational or philosophical.

Consumers of services would be clustered together often sitting idling by. At prescribed periods these people would move around to classes, stations or offices to get treated, served or counseled.

Interaction between staff and consumers would be structured and predictable. In most situations, policies and procedures guide and dictate the actions. Most of the important services happen between 9:00 a.m. and 5:00 p.m. when the more important people (administrators, supervisors and managers) are on duty. Off-hours are the domain of the aides and maintenance staff.

The general intent of the services is to enhance skills or an opportunity to earn modest (or adjusted) wages or to learn how to get along in the world. Any of these alternatives is guided by a goal or service plan that is developed by the experts for the consumer. Clearly, services are designed to fix or protect.

PLANNING / EVALUATION

These activities are vital to any viable organizations, but often are afterthoughts for human services organizations. Usually, agencies make noble attempts to logically plan and look forward, but more often than not, real planning happens in a crisis mode. That is, something occurs that pushes the agency to do some quick planning, but the foresight and systems analysis necessary to good planning is not timely.

On the evaluation side, many human service organizations I know will review their actions and outcomes, but rarely in a formal sense. Those evaluations that do occur are ones that are mandated by funding sources. These reviews, however, are conducted primarily out of the prevailing focus and paradigm.

These seven observations, though not scientifically re-searched, offer a perspective on the current state of human services for persons with disabilities. Most programs I have visited are dedicated and committed organizations. They care about their clients, and lament about the poor outcomes. Yet, as stated earlier, the poor outcomes might be related to the focus and approach and often the organization is lost in its own paradigm. Not only do we need to inspect our services, but we should always be testing the effectiveness to our paradigm. *Interdependence* attempts to articulate a new way to proceed in this process.

In review of all this, three questions have emerged. One is, why have our human services taken on a very similar and predictable face, in spite of the diversity of needs of clients? Two: why have we not had better success in our services? And three: what kinds of new innovations will help us consider necessary changes?

These are not simple questions, but in review of this history of services and our current state, they beg answers. As I reflect on human services today, I have become interested in the foundation that has created the scenes described in these seven basic features. Even though there is a detailed historical per-spective on the development of human services (Bowe, 1978; Wolfensberger, 1971), I feel that there are four prevailing paradigms that converge from this history. These paradigms must be inspected.

MAJOR HUMAN SERVICE PARADIGMS

All organizations are developed from basic roots and vision tied to a body of knowledge that is related to the nature of their business. For example, the banking industry has its roots with economics and capitalistic paradigms. These themes guide the nature and actions of the business that are essential to survival and success.

On the other hand, the church does its business predicated on a basic theology tempered by specifics of the sect. These roots offer a foundation for the routine of its service and a springboard to answer newly-formed questions.

Both types of activities, the church and the bank, are confronted by new pressures and challenges as times and conditions change. The church for example, is confronted by new and complex ethical questions related to life and death as we learn more about the human condition. When life begins, or ends, have become nebulous questions when complexed by life-support equipment and abortion aspects.

As each new day brings adjustments to our questions, the fabric of our paradigms gets renewed challenges. Some of these questions cause us to more deeply explore the roots of our paradigms.

Same too, with human services. As new and complex questions are raised, all of us associated with human services must look inward. As I have been called to do this, I have attempted to articulate the paradigmatic roots of human services. Although there might be some overlap, the four basic paradigms, I believe, that converge to form a human service approach today, are:

- ❖ Medical paradigm
- ❖ Educational paradigm
- ❖ Economic paradigm
- ❖ Maintenance paradigm

Each of these paradigms have specific aspects, but as you read through them, you will notice some common threads. Each will be reviewed separately and then synthesized.

Medical Paradigm

The most influential roots in a general human services paradigm is driven by the medical model. This approach is so powerful and deeply embedded that of its influence is subtle or unconscious. The medical paradigm has grown out of the application of science to the well being of man, and for most of us, is beyond question or challenge. As it has grown and developed, the medical paradigm has some key tenets that set it apart.

One general way that I will review all four paradigms is to use a format that reviews important factors. This approach was initiated by Gerben DeJong (1978), and it is a vivid way to explore paradigms. It reviews how the problem is defined, where the problem rests, what actions have evolved, who has the power, and the intended goal or outcome. Consider this format (See Figure 1) in review of the medical paradigm:

Fig. 1

Medical Paradigms
The Problem — Person with condition Core of Problem — In the person Actions of Paradigm — Classify/congregate/treat Power Person — Expert (doctor) Goal of Paradigm — Fix/heal/change

Since the medical paradigm is so persuasive in human services, we need a closer look to reveal powerful patterns. Culled from the work of Irv Zolla (1986) listed out are some commonly identified patterns:

❖ The professional/physician is the expert and in charge of care or treatment.
❖ Care/treatment is administered through a chain of authority.
❖ The person who receives treatment is labeled (called a patient) and is expected to cooperate.
❖ The main purpose of entry to the paradigm is to restore or fix the person to fit in.
❖ The ailment that brings the person to the paradigm is labeled via a diagnosis.
❖ Literature and research is done and utilized in understanding the specific features of the ailment.
❖ The patient is usually offset and congregated with other like situations.
❖ Most options for control are held by the expert or representative of the paradigm.
❖ Usually the ailment is overshadowed through the therapeutic approach.
❖ The ailment can only be treated by the expert or their agent.
❖ Usually the expert has some credentials or license to treat the ailment.
❖ The patient is exempt from any real responsibility.
❖ Most aspects of the ailment are treated in separate and distinct facilities designed for the ailment.

If you think for a moment about the service you run, work in, or associated with as a family member or consumer, these tenants should not be so far removed. Certainly, there are some differences in traditional medicine, but the drapings of these principles are present in most human service systems I have come to know.

If we look a little deeper at the medical paradigm, there are other key points worth our review. These are:

DEFICIENT ORIENTATION

Without question, medical paradigms focus on what is wrong with the person. Think about the first question the physician asks when a patient enters for an appointment or exam. "What seems to be your problem?" Or, "Tell me where it hurts." In classical medical situations, these questions are essential. In human services, and especially in community based human services, this orientation to deficits is clearly a manifestation of the expert wanting to fix the sick person.

This propensity to stay focused on deficits was driven home to me in a recent workshop I attended designed to sensitize. There were about 20 of us in the session and I only knew a few others in attendance. The workshop leader asked us to get out a sheet of paper after we initially sat down. Of course, as creatures of the banking concept of education, (teacher narrates, students listen) we quickly complied.

He then asked us to write down five things we liked about ourselves and proud were of. No problem for me, I have plenty, and so I jotted away.

Then he asked us to get out another sheet and to record the five things about us that we were uncomfortable about, things we were not proud of and would rather keep quiet. Somewhat suspicious, I complied.

Next, he asked us to pass our positive lists to our right. I beamed, always happy to share my good stuff.

Then the inevitable, "pass the negatives to the left."

"Why?"

"Pass them to the left, don't question the teacher." And so we did.

Now, person to the right of Al Condeluci, introduce this good man. Smiles and accolades.

NOW, PERSON TO THE LEFT OF AL CONDELUCI, INTRODUCE THIS PROBLEMED MAN....As I shrunk in horror, this sadist to my left said it all. Didn't miss one point. All my dirty linen for this roomful of strangers to hear.

Talk about embarrassment! Yet in most human services, this is exactly how we introduce, relate to, or discuss the people that we serve. Most every staffing we conduct is deficit oriented.

I recently sat in a staffing where there were 17 credentialed experts and the client. Each specialist painstakingly articulated problem after problem. Half way through the ordeal, I had to appeal. As I tried to make my points about deficits these experts just looked at me blankly. Some shook their heads as if I really didn't understand.

In another example, after a workshop I conducted on inter-dependence, a staff member from a well-known national pro-gram that specializes in head injury rehabilitation asked for some clarification. She told me of a practice in her program where the program participants start every day with a "realty session." Here, all members of the group let a selected focus person know all of his faults. This staff member said that the sessions get so explosive that the focus person often ends up in tears.

Now, I don't profess to be the last word on things, but somehow I can see no positive conclusion to such practices. Why do we have this love affair with deficits?

CAUSE AND EFFECT

Since medical paradigms are scientific in nature, they usually function from a point of cause and effect. That is, as the paradigm prompts a study and analysis of the ailment, it is drawn to make predictions about what to expect.

In head injury rehabilitation, this might play out by looking at an MRI (this is a type of x-ray that shows the brain and points of damage) and seeing that the frontal lobe is damaged. The automatic prediction is that the effect of the damage will result in some executive thinking difficulty. Cause — damage to frontal lobe; effect — problems in executive thinking. This association is in all the books.

Now, this focus on predictability is not negative in and of itself. Indeed, people predict all the time. The drive to have some association from what we know to what might be, is uniquely human and one of our great attributes. Many times it is a desirable energy. What might be, problematic, however, is when the prediction, especially when it is a negative or deviant one, is then expected and anticipated by everyone around the person with a disability.

Earlier, we reviewed role expectation leading to role behavior. When everyone expects something negative to occur, often it does or will. The old self-fulfilling prophecy.

As I think more about the negative potential of cause and effect, I am reminded of a situation that occurred to me as a teenager. It was my first day of English class when I was going into 8th grade. Like most kids on the first day I was apprehensive and upon entering my English class I sat in the back of the room.

My teacher, a massive lady, started class by going down the roster to see who she had. Three or four names into the list she came to mine, and hesitated. Then she bellowed, "CONDELUCI!!!"

The room fell silent, including me. She screamed again, this time louder and more direct, enunciating each syllable, "CON-DA-LOU-SEE!!!!!"

At this point, one of my buddies, more relieved it was me rather that him, tapped me on the shoulder. I meekly raised my hand, "Here," I whispered.

Scanning the room she spotted me in the back. "GET UP HERE!!!"

Now, I was no angel in those years, but clearly on this day I had not done anything wrong; hell, we had just entered the room. Slowly I rose and started to the front of the room.

Finding a vacant seat in the front, she pointed to it, and I obediently sat in it. She then approached me and getting her face in mine, more intimately than any Drill Sergeant, slowly said, "Last year I had your cousin, Ronnie, in my class, and you Condeluci's are not going to do this to me any more!!!"

By this point, she was manic. The veins in her neck bulging, and my eyes, wide as saucers. There I was, set up in front of my peers no less. Sure, I am a Condeluci, but a problem Condeluci? Cause and effect; a Condeluci and a problem.

My mind raced, and as this massive lady turned back to the blackboard, I did what any red-blooded, problem Condeluci should do...I boldly asserted my middle finger, and said those two infamous words. You know, the ones that start with F and Y.

Not to draw out this story, but the results were one suspended problem Condeluci all on the first day of school.

I understand the importance of prediction based on cause and effect. I also know that at times prediction can go too far, be imprecise, or just plain wrong. I also know that at times a label or determination based on prediction might set a stage of expectation that can lead to the predicted behavior, and in these cases it may be the expert who creates the deviant behavior.

This concept of problems that might be caused by the expert is illuminated by Ivan Illich (1976), in his seminal book, *Medical Nemesis*. In this work, Illich introduces the term, "iatrogenesis" which literally means, physician produced (iatro-Gr. physician, gennan-Gr. to produce). By iatrogenesis, Illich means that physicians (and other agents of the medical paradigm) can create problems as great as those that they heal. He states:

> *Although almost everyone believes that at least one of his friends would not be alive and well except for the skill of a doctor, there is in fact no evidence of any direct relationship between this mutation of sickness and the so called progress of medicine. The changes are dependent variables of political and technological transformations, which in turn are reflected in what doctors do and say; they are not significantly related to the activities that require the preparation, status, and costly equipment in which the health professions take pride. In addition, an expanding proportion of the new burden of disease of the last fifteen years is itself the result of medical intervention in favor of people who are or might become sick. It is doctor-made or iatrogenic.*

After a century of pursuit of medical utopia, and contrary to current conventional wisdom, medical services have not been important in producing the changes in life expectancy that have occurred. A vast amount of contemporary clinical care is incidental to the curing of disease, but the damage done by medicine to the health of individuals and populations is very significant. These facts are obvious, well documented, and well repressed:

... *Awe-inspiring medical technology has combined with egalitarian rhetoric to create the impression that contemporary medicine is highly effective.*
... *The pain, dysfunction, disability, and anguish resulting from technical medical intervention now rival the morbidity due to traffic and industrial accidents and even war-related activities, and make the impact of medicine one of the most rapidly spreading epidemics of our time. Among murderous institutional torts, only modern malnutrition injures more people than iatrogenic disease in its various manifestations.*
... *Medicines have always been potentially poisonous, but their unwanted side effects have increased with their power and widespread use. Every twenty-four to thirty-six hours, from 50 to 80 percent of adults in the United States and the United Kingdom swallow a medically prescribed chemical. Some take the wrong drug, others get an old or contaminated batch, and others a counterfeit; others take several drugs in dangerous combinations; and still others receive injections with improperly sterilized syringes.*

Illich's thesis, is that the medical paradigm is so powerful that it is rarely questioned. Further, since sickness is tied in so closely to life and death, those agents who purport to heal, thus save lives, attain God-like levels in society. How could we ever question them?

To underscore this point, there is a familiar tale about the physician who dies and upon reaching the gates of Heaven is appalled by the long line to get in. Trying to pull rank, he sees a guardian angel and asks if, as a physician, there is any way he can jump line and move closer to the front. The guardian angel says no, and the physician waits his turn in line for what seems like hours. Just before he reaches the gate, a very angelic looking man with a stethoscope and medical bag jumps line and gets in front. Annoyed, the physician summons the guardian angel and says, "What's the deal?". I asked an hour ago if I could jump line and you said no. Then up walks this other doctor and gets right in the gate." The guardian angel replies, "That's no doctor, its just God — he likes to pretend he's a doctor."

Time-worn, this joke illustrates the strength and dominance of the medical paradigm in everyday life. To this point, and related to the aspect of cause and effect, often when the physician says something is so, most lay people believe it is so.

In disability issues, or other areas that are not always scientifically precise, these proclamations can be harmful. I know of numerous situations where families or people with disabilities have been given intense cause and effect information that has been wrong and harmful. The plain and simple truth is that in many situations the medical people just don't know.

Even when medical people admit that they don't know, often the family or person with a disability is so conditioned to believe and hang on the doctor's every word, they mis-hear, or mis-perceive information. Many studies have documented the power of the denial stage early in trauma. Probably the best known review of peoples' readiness to really hear professional help after trauma is *On Death and Dying*, by Elizabeth Kubler-Ross, (1975). In her work, Kubler-Ross suggests that in the early stage of trauma, both the individual who is sick and their family are in a state of denial. At this point, often people cannot rationally hear.

In either way, there can be negative consequences in this issue of cause and effect. All of us who might relate to people who have been devalued, for whatever reason, would do well to recognize this issue and practice with caution.

This aspect of cause and effect and iatrogenic activity is brought home to human services in a recent paper penned by John McKnight (1989), titled, *Do No Harm: A Policymaker's Guide to Evaluating Human Services and Their Alternatives.* In this work, McKnight suggests that every type of treatment or intervention has both positive and negative aspects. Often, however, since human services are not seen to be as serious or scientific as hard medical interventions, there is a tendency to downplay potential iatrogenic consequences. Quite simply, most community-based human services are seen as doing no harm, especially since it is all well intentioned. Yet they can and do.

When I read McKnight's thesis I was reminded of a recent experience I had in a McDonald's restaurant. I stopped by with my children for a quick meal one Saturday, and while sitting down with our burgers, I noticed a van with some writing on the side pull in the parking lot. Then they entered.

First the lead staff came in. Next, four nicely dressed, but shuffling people followed. Finally, the last staff brought up the rear. I immediately had the image of two shepherds with their flock.

They sat down near us and the two shepherds got things set up and took orders. They went for the meals and returned to oversee lunch. I couldn't help notice that people had noticed. I heard the hushed voices of parents telling children not to stare. That these people are "crippled."

As I saw this unfold, I noted that there was both good and bad aspects to this community outing. I'm sure the staff felt that this was a nice day out in the community, and certainly there are some good aspects about getting out.

On the other hand, however, there were some real negative images about this outing. People who appear strange, clustered together, shepherds hovering over them, a well marked van that announced their deviance, their apparent inability to order, even with the simple McDonald's menu, all these things, in effect were iatrogenic.

TREATMENT FROM A DIAGNOSIS

Most people who are disenfranchised, have some diagnosis that sets them apart from the norm. This diagnosis defines the parameters of the deviance, and gives the expert some anchor to understanding their ailment.

Touching on both previous points, the diagnosis is usually riddled with deficits and deviance that make the person strange or special. It also offers a starting point for cause and effect predictions. Its other manifestation, however, is found in the shear power of the labeling process. Once a label is ascribed, an entire parade of stereotypes follow.

To this point, Biklen and Knoll (1987), in *Community Integration for People with Severe Disabilities*, wrote:

> ...*While a disability is but one of many personal qualities - such as stature, hair color, geographic origin, race, and sex - it is frequently a basis for negative evaluation. People with disabilities find themselves given labels such as mentally retarded, brain injured, deaf, blind, emotionally disturbed, mentally ill, autistic or learning disabled. Occasionally, these labels become epithets: "What are you, blind?" "It's like the blind leading the blind." "Retard." "What are you, deaf?" For severely disabled people, there is the term "vegetable." While professionals will sometimes make the case for the social utility of classifications and labeling - for example, to decide who needs special school or clinic services, or economic subsidies - we cannot help wondering why such services cannot be provided without subjecting people to disability labels.*

When you think of it, the labelling process creates an entire tone about the person. It's set up to expect certain things from the labeled person, based on what you know or understand about the label. For most disenfranchised people, what we know or perceive about them is usually negative. To this extent, we begin to look for the problems.

A study in Canada recently confirmed the debilitating effects of labeling (Lord & Farlow, 1990). In a detailed review of 38 people with devaluing labels they stated:

Our data shows that people who have been labeled because of disability or poverty have generally experienced extended periods of powerlessness in their lives as a result of segregation, prolonged dependency and failures in community support services...

Moreover, as one key informant emphasized, 'Once a person is labeled, professionals only see the person's problems...It is then impossible for the person to escape from the system's definition of them.

On a more personal note, think about labelling experiences that may have happened to you; especially a label you did not like, or was not very complimentary. It might have been a nickname or a way someone described you. These labels were probably hurtful to you, and you couldn't wait for the time you could escape the image. Now think about people who cannot escape.

A number of years ago, at my agency, the issue of labels was hotly examined. People could understand the intellectual discussion about the stigmatic nature of labels, but justified their use of labels from the perspective that they were not using them in a harmful way. As if their intentions exonerated them from the community mythology of the label. Others, followed Biklen and Knoll's point, that the label was merely a social description needed for reports and proposals. Still others justified labels from the perspective that we are all labeled. They said that their lawyer calls them client and they don't get mad at the label.

Now all of these points are veiled. We really don't need labels. We use them because they are convenient, simpler for us, and are sanctioned by the medical paradigm. The bottom line, however, is that they are not needed. They perpetuate group images, cast people into powerful stereotypes, and lead way to role expectation and the iatrogenic aspects of cause and effect. Let's be rid of them, lest we do more harm.

THE "SICK ROLE"

Perhaps the most powerful manifestation of the medical paradigm is found in review of the concept of the sick role. Here the person is given the authority to be sick and to surrender autonomy to the agent of the paradigm so that he can be made better.

However, Illich points out that it is the paradigm that defines what is well and what is sick. Further, only the paradigm can decide if sickness has indeed turned into wellness. It sets the rules, decides who fits, determines what the outcomes should be, establishes its own mechanism to measure success, and then retains authority to proclaim wellness.

This notion of the sick role creates a sense of learned helplessness. As the devalued person is continually positioned in the sick role, he not only accepts the phenomena, but begins to learn how to be helpless. I recall an arrangement I had with a fellow we supported who had some memory challenges. To build on his capacities, I had him call me every Wednesday to discuss things and plan out activities.

Things went well for a few weeks, and then one Tuesday, he called. As we talked, I reminded him that this was not our regularly scheduled day to talk. After some silence he said: "Well what did you expect, I'm brain damaged and I have a memory impairment." This was an example, I believe, of learned helplessness.

Another manifestation of the sick role rests with the authority to define the problem. In the medical paradigm, the problem is always defined by the expert or the authority. Rarely does the patient get to define his ailment. The expert will ask for symptoms, but will retain the right and privilege to render a diagnosis. Certainly this makes sense when we are dealing with various types of diseases, but when we shift to consider most of the challenges facing people with disability, this phenomena can create devaluation.

Although we know that the ability to define our own situations is a powerful component of empowerment, the medical community still maintains its posture that the expert, not the consumer, knows best. (Dunst, Trivete, & Deal, 1988). This perspective is not only disempowering, but at times, downright arrogant.

The key point for me in this concept of the sick role rests with the surrendering of power to the authority. To a certain extent, this is giving away and giving up. It also says that the sick are really not good, until they can be like the well. This becomes incredibly vexing when the ailment is one that cannot be totally fixed, such as in brain damage, or other types of permanent disabilities. Can these people ever be well? Further, once a person surrenders, how can he ever get back full power and authority, especially if it is never really regained until the person can be like the well? Most recent work on the concept of empowerment, which is linked to interdependence, stress that the first stage to regaining control in one's life is gaining back the right to define the problem.

PATIENT MUST ADAPT OR ADJUST

Another strong point of the medical paradigm is found in the goal of fixing people. That is, the onus for change rests squarely on the shoulders of the patient. It is he or she who must change, adapt, or adjust to the existing world. If the person cannot walk, talk, or act like the rest of society as he enters the medical paradigm, then the charge is to make this happen for the person. Countless hundreds of medical paradigm agents work tirelessly toward this goal almost regardless of the will of the person with a disability.

When I think of this aspect of the medical paradigm, I think of a friend of mine from Boston, who a few years ago, sustained a spinal cord injury in an auto accident. After he was medically stabilized, he spent 18 months in a rehabilitation hospital with emphasis on learning his daily living activities. Hundreds of hours of costly therapeutic time was spent teaching him how to dress himself in an effort to become "independent."

After all this effort, upon discharge, indeed he was able to dress himself. Lo and behold, it took him two hours to get dressed by himself in the morning. TWO HOURS! And after all this effort, he hardly had energy left for anything else.

Now he wonders, and so do I, why all the time, money and effort were spent on a goal, that in and of itself, is not functional for his real need. In his thinking, if the same money spent over the course of his ADL rehabilitation was used to create an attendant service pool, he could have had an attendant take 30 minutes in the morning to dress him and like you or me, be off to his day, and the funding could have lasted his whole projected lifetime!

Certainly dressing oneself is important, but in the case of my friend, it was seen as the only way to prepare him for independence. It implied that any adjusting or changing necessary to make this happen was up to him. The paradigm did not allow for any exploration of how other things might change to promote an independence for him.

This idea of adjusting or changing is particularly challenging, when a person's situation is so severe or permanent that change or adjustment is impossible. These kinds of situations in the medical paradigm create a vexing challenge. This is a situation that totally defies the paradigms propensity to deal effectively. These challenges are also the stuff that push a paradigm shift. In cases of severe and permanent disabilities, the medical paradigm is not capable of meeting the challenge.

CLINICAL EFFICACY

A final factor that deeply roots the medical paradigm is found in what I call *clinical efficacy*. This term relates to the strong drive that medical paradigm clinicians have to validate their practice.

This concept is not hard to appreciate, considering that most agents of the medical paradigm must have a license or some sort of sanction to practice. To achieve this, these people must put in countless hours of schooling and tutelage under the direction of those thought to be masters. Remember, however, that these masters are the guardians of the paradigm. They are rewarded and validated by the paradigm, so it should not be difficult to understand their protection and defense. Thus newcomers to the paradigm are indoctrinated and held accountable to the tenants.

Further, along with the time it takes to gain license, newcomers to the paradigm usually must invest a good deal of money. This might come in the form of tuition, dues, certification, testing, books or journals needed, equipment and other associated paraphernalia. After all this investment of time and money, most agents of the medical paradigm do not want to have their roots questioned or tested.

Often, when I give talks or workshops on this type of review of the medical paradigm, I get interesting reactions from medical professionals. Some are engaged by the review and basically embrace the concepts. Others, however, become defensive and angry at the implication that medical treatment might have some iatrogenic aspects.

I remember one neuropsychologist in particular who approached me after a keynote speech before a large medically allied group. "Shame on you for saying the things you did about medicine. There are many young and impressionable clinicians here who might believe what you say," she said in a scolding fashion.

Another talk in Canada found me sharing the podium with a well-known psychiatrist. After his relatively bland and traditional review of rehabilitation, I shared concepts about interdependence that challenged the medical paradigm. My comments ignited the audience, and during the question and answer period, the psychiatrist was somewhat under attack. At the close of the session, he refused to shake my hand. Challenging paradigms is not the best way to win friends.

Educational Paradigm

Educational paradigms refer to the structure and underpinnings of the way people are educated. Although we often think of education in relationship to children, educational paradigms refer to all types of educational settings. To this extent, we need to consider educational settings not only from the classic grade school, high school and college levels, but related to business, trade, and upgrading of skills as well. The area of rehabilitation as an educational paradigm falls into this later scheme.

Again, for consistency, consider the educational paradigm (See Figure 2) off the five aforementioned review factors:

Fig. 2

Educational Paradigm

The Problem — Student doesn't know
Core of Problem — In student's ability
Actions of Paradigm — Classify/congregate/teach
Power Person — Teacher
Goals of Paradigm — Student learns new info

In his powerful book, *Pedagogy of the Oppressed*, Paulo Freire (1989), describes and reviews the education paradigm as follows:

❖ The teacher teaches and the students are taught;
❖ The teacher knows everything and the student knows nothing;
❖ The teacher thinks and the students are thought about;
❖ The teacher talks and the students listen — meekly;
❖ The teacher disciplines and the students are disciplined;
❖ The teacher chooses and enforces his choice, and the students comply;
❖ The teacher acts and the students have the illusion of acting through the action of the teacher;
❖ The teacher chooses the program content, and the students (who were not consulted) adapt to it;
❖ The teacher confuses the authority of knowledge with his own personal authority, which he sets in opposition to the freedom of the students;
❖ The teacher is the subject of the learning process, while the pupils are mere objects.

Another educator who has been critical of the educational paradigm was Myles Horton (1989). The founder of the Highlander Research and Education Center in Tennessee said:

> *Our educational institutions have a top-down decision making process which insure bureaucratic control. Nothing short of a powerful and sustained people's movement to liberate education will basically change the situations in schools and society.*

Although Horton's work focused on adult education, his thoughts are relevant to all of education. Certainly, most rehabilitation education flows from the adult education model, thus his thoughts seem all that much more germane to interdependence.

Both Horton's and Freire's review of the educational paradigm have solid relevance to human services, especially those that are community based. I have been in countless programs around the country that have a pedagogical format and are conducted out of an educational paradigm. Much like medical models, these educational paradigms have some key tenants that we must be conscious of. These are:

THE PROBLEM

In the educational paradigm, the problem in question is that the student lacks certain knowledge. This approach assumes that the student has some knowledge, but lacks key information in comparison to other people in the person's age range. These homogeneous comparisons are critical to the educational paradigm. It uses all types of tests and national norms to establish a baseline. If the person in question is below the baseline, they are usually devalued and, at times, punished by the system.

On the other hand, students who are above the norm, although not devalued, are often not stimulated to the point that is helpful. Yet our educational paradigm continues to promote that children of like age be together for an inordinate amount of time and be constantly compared to each other.

John Gatto, New York City's Teacher of the Year in 1989, stated in his acceptance speech, *Why Schools Don't Educate*:

> It is absurd and anti-life to be part of a system that compels you to sit in confinement with people of exactly the same age and social class. That system effectively cuts you off from the immense diversity of life and the synergy of variety. It cuts you off from your own past and future, sealing you in a continuous present much the same way television does.

Still, the educational paradigm moves forward to promote the banking approach to information. New facts upon new facts are added on to the person, primarily in the quest of irradicating the problem — limited information of the student within parameters of the national norms.

Given this approach of the banking concept, Freire believes that a student can never develop the mode of thinking critically about issues. He states:

> It is not surprising that the banking concept of education regards men as adaptable, manageable beings. The more students work at storing the deposits entrusted to them, the less they develop the critical consciousness which would result from their interven-

tion in the world as transformers of that world. The more completely they accept the passive role imposed upon them, the more they tend simply to adapt to the world as it is and to the fragmented view of reality deposited in them.

CORE OF THE PROBLEM

If the problem of the educational paradigm is limited information, the source of the problem rests in the fact that the student doesn't know the information. To this extent, the emanation of the problem rests with the student. Often it is perceived that the student is naive, ignorant, or just not motivated to want to acquire new information. In this analysis, if the student does not learn, it is primarily his fault.

Thus when educational experts come together to review their failures, they focus most time and attention on how to motivate, or entice the student to pick up the new information. To this point Gatto states:

> *Experts in education have never been right; their solutions are expensive, self serving, and always involve further centralization. Enough.*

These actions are clearly efforts to protect the existing paradigm.

ACTIONS OF THE PARADIGM

Teacher dominance

As Freire suggests, the kings of educational paradigms are the teachers. They are clearly in control, and all action revolves around them. From pre-school situations to doctoral work, the teacher reigns supreme. Yet, as most of us would agree, there have probably been times when the teacher was inept, unprepared, or just plain wrong. In these situations, however, if challenged at all, the loser was probably the student.

Often, this teacher domination is operational through obedience. That is, the student who obeys the teacher is rewarded. The ones who do not are punished. This punishment can run the gamut from ridicule or banishment to corporal punishment. The lessons of obedience are often set early and in powerful ways.

I can remember my first day in first grade. Like most six-year olds, we were energized, though certainly not socialized or conditioned to the ways of school. Then we met Miss O.

Though average-sized, Miss O took her job of introduction to obedience seriously and in a physical way. On our first day, she set the rules down. "You will sit in your seats quietly. You will listen to what I say. You will only move when I tell you to move. You will... You will not..." All these deep and powerful messages given in drill sergeant cadence to small and vulnerable creatures.

Like most six-year-olds, however, some of our attention spans were shorter than others. Such was the plight of a jumpy kid in my class named Tony. Although he heard Miss O's rules and regulations, the passage of time was his downfall. After only a few minutes of the setting of the rules, Tony, driven by curiosity, got from his seat and meandered to the window.

Miss O, when she saw the infraction, seemingly could not believe her eyes. She followed Tony to the window and cleared her throat behind him. Tony didn't flinch until Miss O grabbed him by the scruff of the shirt and escorted him back to his seat.

Hovering over him, Miss O proceeded to repeat the rules and regulations, this time with a stronger pitch to her voice. Not ten minutes later, that madman Tony was up again and off to the window.

Now Miss O was a veteran of many first day, first grade situations. She knew the importance of dealing with this type of challenge quickly.

Without any noise or effort Miss O grabbed Tony, again by the scruff of the shirt, but this time lifting him off his feet, and using only one hand, she hauled him to the front of the room. With her foot, she nudged the trash can from underneath her desk, and then firmly and cleanly she stuffed Tony into the trash can.

With only Tony's head and feet showing from the can, 30 dumbfounded six-year-olds learned our first pedagogical lesson of obedience, domination, and oppression.

Power Persons

The educational paradigm mandates that teachers teach and students are taught. This basic notion of passivity suggests that the students have nothing to offer. Further, what they do offer is gauged or judged by the teacher according to the standards they have set.

Sometimes, these standards are obvious such as with mathematics or hard sciences. In most of these cases, there really is only one answer. But in many other things, the notion of standards is an arbitrary venture. In cases such as writing, or art, or philosophy, the teacher can often set a standard that may be debatable to an adult observer, but never to the student.

As these issues of student passivity take hold, many students learn the big lessons of the paradigm: listen, obey and never challenge. This approach continues well into college and graduate school. I remember clearly the advice of a post graduate instructor when he told me, "Al, Wait until you get your Ph.D., and then ruffle all the feathers you want." From first grade to a university Ph.D., obedience and passivity does pay off.

Goal of Paradigm

In educational settings, the goal is a changed or enlightened student, capable of repeating the information or solving the problems posed by the teacher. This is usually gauged by passage of a test, or achieving a certain level in comparison with other like people, according to some national norm.

A further gauge of success is determined by the teacher or expert in a review of the performance of the student. The expert and agent of the paradigm determines who does and does not pass.

The obvious point is that the student must demonstrate some change or mastery over a subject or topic. If they cannot, they are considered failures and must repeat the course. In most cases, this failure is humiliating and belittling. Often it is the first step to turning off persons to the very goal considered important to the paradigm. That is, if having people value and pursue education is a goal of the paradigm, failing people is not a way to achieve this goal.

And so, the educational paradigm looms as equally powerful. With a microscopic focus it follows the lead of the medical paradigm to identify the student as the problem, have experts define the actions, and attempts to fix or change the students.

With this analysis under our belts, let's now turn to the economic paradigm.

Economic Paradigm

A third major approach that has impact and relevance to human services is found in the economic paradigm. This model relates primarily to the value exchange usually associated with goods, services, or money.

Like the two previous paradigms, the economic paradigm is deep-rooted and prominent in our western culture. Given our capitalistic dominance and our love affair with money, this paradigm deals with the potential for performance and value of skills.

Quite simply, it mixes the Darwinian theory with the protestant work ethic to create a strong paradigm that has no room for people who have a disability. Some key features of the economic paradigm are better understood with our overview shown in Figure 3.

Fig. 3

Economic Paradigm
The Problem — Person can't earn living Core of Problem — In person's incapabilities Actions of Paradigm — Assess/train/place/subsidize Power Person — The vocational expert/attorney Goal of Paradigm — Find job/settlement

PROBLEM

The focus of the economic paradigm relates primarily to the ability, or inability to get or hold a job that contributes to the personal economy of the individual or family. In this perspective, all members of the family must contribute to the economic well-being of the family. Consequently, like the pioneer/farm families we see in the movies or read about, all members must do their share. This contribution could be direct, like a paycheck, or indirect such as keeping the home front viable while others bring home the paycheck.

When the economic paradigm meets people with disabilities, they are sized up as to the deficits that may interfere with the process of economy. That is, the person is assessed as to the ability or inability to produce, contribute or hold a job. Given the influence of the aforementioned medical paradigm, these assessments look primarily at what is wrong with the person to prevent them from being productive or holding a job.

Today, in the human service world that surrounds disability, a battery of tests and surveys attempts to identify and predict the economic potential of its clients. These tests look at aptitude, interests, skills, education, and deficits. It is mostly the deficits, however, that cast a shadow on the plan that is set up for the individual.

CORE OF PROBLEM

As we look closer at the inner dimensions of economic paradigm, there seems to be a strong and stereotypic relationship between success and performance. That is, if people have physical and cognitive skills and abilities to perform, then they will probably be successful economically.

The reverse of this then, is the less physical and cognitive skills one has, the less economic potential. The stereotypic message is, when an employer looks to hire a person, they will select the most skillful. Greater the skills, the more value to the company. Further, the more skills and potential, the more value the person will have to the human service agency as well. This is due to the potential success the person brings to the rehabilitation agency in showing that they can indeed help the "handicapped."

This close tie between skills and value is vital to understanding the economic model. The more skills one has, the further they will get economically. It then seems natural to promote the acquisition of skills as the secret to success. Thus, if the person has deficits that might be in the way of skill acquisition, we must know these deficits, and eradicate them.

Another associated dimension is between quantity of work and the value ascribed to the person who can deliver more. This element of quantity is sometimes related to strength, dexterity, memory, or what we call intelligence. People with stronger levels in these areas will be more valuable because they can seemingly deliver more.

A subdivision of quantity is speed of delivery. This means that often quantity is affected by the speed in which the goods can be delivered. Indeed, in western culture we place great value on speed on almost all fronts. The person who can read fast, or talk fast, or think fast is valued. The speed wars in our society have even played out with pizza delivery. This love affair with speed creates a formidable obstacle to the person who is slow or less efficient.

ACTIONS OF THE PARADIGM

Given the problem and its core, the economic paradigm has etched out some actions specifically related to disability. These are:

Assessment of skills

Before individuals are admitted to any situation that has economic relevance, they must be assessed as to their skill and ability to participate. These assessments look primarily at the elements usually associated with success in the chosen area. The elements that the person cannot perform are then targeted to be taught.

In this area of assessment, it is important to note that often those who guide people to certain jobs or careers may be biased. That is, they might have some preset judgement of the individual based on the stereotypes that have been ingested.

This phenomena happens in all walks of life, but nowhere does it seem to be more vivid than in the area of disability. Time and time again, the experts at the core of economic paradigms push people with certain disabilities toward job areas thought to be best with disability groups. Classic areas are:

Mental Retardation	-custodian -dishwasher -busboy
Visual Disability	-broommaker -cafeteria vendor
Auditory Disability	-loud factory -printer
Brain Injury	-repetitive work -microfilm work
Cord Injury	-counselor -disability advocate -accountant

Clearly, some people request these areas, and some may be very good at them. The point is, that the biases of those who guide, counselors, teachers, parents, or friends can be so influenced by the economic paradigm, they unconsciously fall into its clutches.

Training

Once the assessment is complete, usually the individual will be guided to a training program associated with the job selected or deficits that need remedial action in order to obtain the job. For most people with disabilities, the remedial route is the one often followed. The paradigm demands that these problems be fixed before the person can or should enter the job or vocation planned.

This trend toward remediation has created an entire human service industry with the sole purpose of getting people with disabilities ready to enter some type of work. We have pre-work skill training, cognitive remediation, pre-vocational training, work hardening, work practice, volunteer work, and numerous others, all with the goal of getting people ready for work.

To this point, Thomas Bellamy et al. (1988) in their book, *Supported Employment*, stated:

> *If an individual with a severe disability entered the continuum in a day-activity program and progressed through the continuum at the estimated average rate, he or she would spend 37 years preparing for a work-activity center, another 10 years in such a center before moving to a workshop or a job, and 9 more years in a regular program workshop. In other words, an individual who entered this continuum upon completing school at age 21 would begin his or her first job at age 77.*

When you pause to reflect on these trends, the idea of remediation does seem plausible from the context of the economic paradigm. If the sheer ability to work at all is tied to performance, then the need for remediation, for those who do not seem capable, is natural. Yet, in light of Bellamy's suggestion, most people with disabilities who are in pre-vocational settings never get to work situations, in spite of all the remediation. The data is showing clearly that people are not getting jobs, or once gotten, not holding jobs. The reality is that remediation doesn't work.

Job Placement

Another action within the economic paradigm is to find people jobs. In the human service industry, this agenda gets played out in job placement activities.

Job placement is the formal stage of economic re-engagement for people who have been disenfranchised from the community. It endeavors to find jobs for people within the area of their aptitude or training. It is important to note, however, the area of job placement in the disability perspective has grown into a mandate and specialty.

The Rehabilitation Act, from which all state-supported vocational rehabilitation activities operate, has included job placement as a mandated service since its inception. All public and many private vocational rehabilitation services make job placement available.

As these programs have developed, however, the thrust has become a charity type of approach. That is, many people with disabilities are marketed by job placement specialists, much as one might market a commodity.

I can recall a recent situation where I made a pitch to a local hospital to consider hiring a woman I know who has a head injury. Working with her, we positioned her capabilities in a positive way and finally the hospital decided to take a chance on hiring her. She did such a good job for them that within three months they called us back to request "a few more of those type of people."

That experience was a wake-up call to my consciousness. As I thought about the experience, my first inclination was to get angry at the hospital. How could they have reacted so crassly as to consider my friend one of "those type of people?" With further review, however, I realized that it really wasn't the fault of the hospital at all. Sure, they had responded crassly, but the hospital really did nothing more than parrot the image I had created. I sold them a commodity, and they acted accordingly. The real culprit, in my review, was me.

Workshops and programs

A final action of the economic paradigm is found in the creation of workshops and programs when job placement fails, or individuals with disabilities are perceived to be so severe that they cannot be employed in real work.

Workshops and programs have become equally proliferated in the human service world. It's as if we have to do something with "these people" and if we cannot place them, then we must provide programs for "them." Given the paradigm's perspective of the limited worth of these people, however, the programs must be economical and austere. This is a powerful notion to ponder.

The paradigm that places increased value on those with potential, places little value on those perceived to have less potential. Thus, the charity image gets further rooted into our system. As this limited value is ascribed to persons with severe disabilities, the programs that are created for them flow from the cloth of heavy congregation, segregation and unbelievably poor staff ratios. In an ironic paradox, those who may need the most support, wind up in programs that provide the least.

I have visited hundreds of programs around the United States and Canada and invariably the ones for the most severely disabled are the most pathetic. Often they are in poorer sections of town, or donated church space. Resources are "hand-me-down" and clients are left to sit in idle, unproductive time.

In some cases, these poor realities have been realized and experts have worked to up-grade conditions. Still, the results of these efforts have been transparent.

I was once in Kansas to do some training. The course was held at a new sheltered workshop and my hosts were quick to give me a grand tour, proud of their new facility. As we moved from section to section I did notice the bright color and sky lights. It was truly an architectural masterpiece. I also noticed, however, the same faces, and idleness and time-wasting that I have observed in countless sheltered workshops around the country. Although this was a pretty facility, it was business as usual in the sheltered workshop industry.

Power Persons

As with the medical and educational paradigms discussed earlier, the economic paradigm is also driven by experts who think they know what is best. In the economic arena, for the most part, the experts are vocational rehabilitation counselors. Usually this group of professionals is the one that makes the initial determination of potential.

Others who can set an economic tone for people with disabilities include special education teachers, counselors, social workers, family, advocates, lawyers, or friends. Regardless, the person with a disability is often spoken for or guided through the process of career/work awareness. Many people with disabilities that I know have felt extremely oppressed by this process. This assumption of control is a direct act of devaluation and a key feature of disempowerment.

As previously mentioned, these experts can make decisions from a number of approaches including stereotypic biases. In fact, this phenomena is certainly not exclusive to disability biases. Other groups, who have been equally oppressed or devalued, are subject to the same treatment, African-Americans and women are two good examples.

Since the days of slavery, certain vocational scripts have been written for African-Americans. Initially the maintenance, custodial, porter, and caretaker positions were the typical vocational opportunities. Today, we see more subtle ways that people of color are economically oppressed. Interesting enough, the typical jobs reserved for people of color are now being increasingly filled by people with disabilities. If I was paranoid, I might think there was some type of "Murphy's Law" that says he who is lowest in value, gets the worst jobs.

Women too, have been similarly type-cast. There are certain jobs that are perceived to be "women's work." Things such as nursing, secretarial, social work, and the like have been almost exclusively scripted for women.

As the women's movement has opened up new opportunities today, women still find themselves caught in an economic web. That is, as women take their rightful place in other types of occupations, they are still held accountable for the smooth flow of the home front. And so, women find themselves responsible to two masters, something that men rarely face. They must keep up the home, the children, and compete in jobs that demand more than a 9:00 to 5:00 schedule.

As I think about this "type-casting," I am inclined to continue the story from my youth. You know, the one about the time I was suspended by falling into the role expectation set for me by my eighth-grade English teacher.

As the story continues, I went home after my suspension to await my fate. My nerves were high, but when I saw my dad and the principal arrive simultaneous at my home that night, I almost lost it. I knew that I had my work cut out trying to explain to my dad, but there was the principal, too! When they entered the house, I was still in my bedroom on the second floor. As they sat down at the kitchen table, I scootched down the top two stairs and strained to hear the muffled conversation.

"Now, Sinbad, your boy is not all that bad. Granted, what he did to Mrs. G was uncalled for, but I have been checking his records. Basically, he's not a bad boy. I'm worried though, that this might be a signal, and have been thinking about his future."

I could then hear bits and pieces of my dad's response and question. "Well, what do you think, Ed? What do the records say? What might be possible for Al?"

By this time, I was down to the middle of the stairway, in almost a comical contortion on the steps, leaning over to hear it all.

"Well, Sinbad, you know his grades aren't all that good. I don't think college is a real good idea. He also doesn't seem to have any real viable skills or talents."

My mind, by now, was racing — no academic skills! No viable talents! Just what was my fate to be?

Then the principal said, "You know, Sinbad, he might do well in construction or cement work. You might want to consider that."

CONSTRUCTION OR CEMENT WORK!! Talk about stereotypes! I might as well have had the map of Italy on my forehead. Everyone knows that construction and cement work are in our genes. Show Italians a trowel, and immediately they run off to the nearest construction site to finish off the cement job.

As I think today of that experience, I have no ill feelings toward my principal. I believe he was caught in the baggage of his day. He had a bias about Italians and it played out in his actions. The point is, these kind of stereotypes are powerful and telling. They can direct and stunt a person's life. They are often unconscious, or subconscious notions, but problematic nonetheless. We need to deeply inspect these trends, they are the stuff that keep people oppressed.

Paradigm goal

The goal of the economic paradigm is to get people jobs so they can have some economic base for participation. In many regards, this goal gets played out in trying to teach, adjust, or change the person in question. If a job cannot be performed, it is due to a deficit manifest in the person, and that's what must change.

Most of the energy and actions of the paradigm are microscopic to the person. The goal is to ultimately promote skills that lead to value, but usually through some way the person can change or adapt. The paradigm demands that people adjust to it. The logical next question is, what about the person who just cannot change or adjust.

As I ponder the economic paradigm goal and this logical question, I remember vividly an experience that occurred a few years ago.

A family I had previously helped with some advocacy work, approached me after the death of their son. They were devastated by his death, which happened when he choked on some food while staying at a local intermediate care facility. Somehow, someway, they needed to respond to his death.

As we met, I suggested we contact a friend of mine who specialized in disability law. Perhaps through legal recourse, this family could find some solace.

As we sat with my friend, she reviewed some documents on this family's son and some photos. He was a handsome lad, just 14 when he died. After looking over the material, my friend paused and looked slowly at the three of us.

She said, "Look, I can take this case and we can take the facility to court, but I need to tell you that I don't think we will win."

The three of us looked quizzically as she continued. "You see, your son was very severely disabled, not able to do anything for himself. A judge or jury will weigh that heavily. They will consider his value.

Again, we looked at each other, then the father said, "His value? What does that have to do with it? Our son is dead."

Now, my friend is a very sensitive and caring person, and a fine lawyer. She responded softly, "I know this is hard to hear, because it is hard for me to say, but the court will consider the value and worth of your son's life and then make some decisions on that. They will probably consider him worth very little. Further, and I know this is hard, but since the state was contributing to his care...." She didn't have to say the rest!

This review of the economic paradigm is not designed to totally disregard the good or positive elements of the paradigm. There are some constructive aspects inherent in the economic model. There are also, as in any paradigm, shortcomings. As we look at interdependence, we need to consciously examine and understand the paradigms that drive human services today, both their good and bad.

Maintenance Paradigm

The final paradigm that I believe is dominant in human services today is the maintenance paradigm. Although elements of this paradigm are visible throughout human services, in rehabilitation this paradigm is most dominant after all the major services have been rendered by the experts, and the person still has not been fixed. Rather than fault the other paradigms (medical, educational and economic) the blame of failure is passed on to the individual, who is ushered into a new paradigm to be taken care of.

A clearer way to understand how these paradigms can work in tandem, and not find major weaknesses with any of them, is to consider a person who might have had a severe head injury. Immediately after injury, the person is labeled a patient and enters the medical paradigm. There, all the major elements discussed earlier occur. Once the person has been saved and stabilized, he is passed on to a medical/educational paradigm to be restored. Usually, this medical/educational level is actualized in rehabilitation services. As the person gets closer to restoration, the economic paradigm is introduced to promote job preparation and, ultimately, job placement. At this point, if all has gone smoothly, the person is discharged and pronounced fixed.

If, however, the person has manifestations from head injury that create more problems than the paradigm can handle, the paradigm must find some way to avoid failure. Enter the maintenance paradigm.

The maintenance paradigm is best understood as a caretaker approach. Another name often ascribed is custodial. It essentially assumes that there is not much hope for improvement for the individual, so maintaining the present functioning level becomes the overall goal. As with the other paradigms we have discussed, the maintenance paradigm can be reviewed as follows:

Fig. 4

Maintenance Paradigm
The Problem — Person needs care Core of Problem — In person's deficits Actions of Paradigm — Congregate/care/control Power Person — Benevolent caretakers Goal of Paradigm — Maintain/prepare for death

PROBLEM

The basic problem presented to the maintenance paradigm, is that the person needs care. Forget fixing, or restoring, or any other type of education. The major thrust is to maintain the person.

Perhaps the best way to get a quick understanding of the maintenance paradigm is to make a visit to your nearest nursing home. It really doesn't matter in what town, community or state. Give or take a few amenities, they are much the same. As you visit, the most common feature is how similar the residents all appear. Regularity and order are important facets of the maintenance paradigm.

When I graduated from college, my first job was in a large geriatric center where clearly the prevailing paradigm was that of maintenance.

I remember how vivid my first impressions, still strong as I reflect back some 21 years. There were over 2,000 residents at this facility, and while touring, I was amazed at how orderly everything was. Corridors were lined with white haired, toothless people, all in "geri-chairs." These devices look much like a barber's chair, with restraints to keep the occupant in place. Most of the "patients," as they were called, looked alike. In fact, the men all wore these grey cotton blazers and special no-skid slippers. Hair cuts and hairdos seemed to be standard order, and at times, it was hard for me to tell who was who. Of course, the fact that I was the social worker assigned to over 500 men, didn't help.

In this setting, and most others like it, the major challenge is to take care of the residents. It is assumed that these folks cannot take care of themselves. At the facility where I worked, almost all daily living tasks were done or closely supervised by staff, no matter the skill or capability of the resident.

CORE OF THE PROBLEM

As with the other paradigms, the problems encountered by the maintenance paradigm rest within the person. It is the fact that the person is elderly, disabled, or sick that has caused them to enter the paradigm.

An important feature to appreciate, however, is the paradigm perceives that these people will probably not get better, or improve in functioning. In fact, the paradigm expects them to deteriorate. There is a powerful sense of hopelessness.

One of the most frustrating aspects of my work in the geriatric center revolved around this notion of hopelessness. Time and time again, I found my efforts to establish more appropriate living arrangements thwarted by a host of paradigm experts who contended that the "patients" just could not do what I was promoting, or that it wasn't worth it. The problems of their age, disability, or condition was too deeply embedded for the experts to let go.

ACTIONS OF THE PARADIGM

Given these perspectives, the actions of the paradigm are few and isolated. The major action, of course, is delivering care to keep those at the point of the paradigm safe and secure. Further, since the value of those who receive services is low, the services must be humble and inexpensive. This is why nursing home staff/resident ratios are so stark. It is not worth it to provide more care than absolutely necessary. The hopelessness factor serves to exacerbate this point.

Driven by these factors, maintenance paradigms, and those experts within these paradigms, are thought to be charitable and benevolent. As mentioned previously in this text, I am always struck by the reaction of friends who learn that I work with people who have disabilities.

Their first assumption is that we are taking care of "them." Next, their notion is that we are special for doing so. I don't kid when I liken the response of many to that of Dana Carvey's church lady on the TV show, "Saturday Night Live," when she says, "Aren't you special!"

As I have read, and understood Wolf Wolfensberger's (1987) perspective on *Deathmaking*, I am inclined to consider another action of the maintenance paradigm; that of preparing the persons in the paradigm for their own death. In "*Deathmaking*," Wolfensberger argues that systems that surround devalued people can unconsciously promote death by withholding services or treating devalued people in such a way so that they are more vulnerable. He defines "deathmaking" as, "any actions or pattern of actions which either directly or indirectly bring about, or hasten, the death of a person or group." Given the hopelessness ascribed to those in the maintenance paradigm, the experts and caretakers often feel it is important to prepare them for the inevitable.

Indeed, it was tragic for me to witness how loved ones close to persons admitted to the geriatric center, slowly withdraw time and attention from their family member. This phenomena is similar to the withdrawal actions described in Kubler-Ross's work (1969). Due to our own fears and shortcomings, we pull back from those we know or perceive to be dying.

IN-CHARGE EXPERTS

Staying true to its microscopic roots, the maintenance paradigm is driven and controlled by expert caretakers. These include nurses, aides, administrators, and geriatric technicians. These people are often trained, and like counterparts from other paradigms discussed, must have some license or certification to hold their jobs. Out of all the paradigms discussed, however, the maintenance paradigm seemingly has the lowest standards.

This is probably because the paradigm participants are the most devalued.

Directly tied to these lowered standards is lower scale of wage. Quite simply, workers in the maintenance paradigm are paid the lowest. Again, this wage differential is clearly related to the extent and "spread" of devaluation. Since those in the maintenance paradigm are "losers," why value or pay paradigm workers decent wage?

Similarly, participants in the maintenance paradigm have even less say about their life situation than those caught in other paradigms. Often they are not consulted about anything that affects their lives. This obvious disregard is a loud signal about who is in charge, and who is important.

PARADIGM GOAL

Quiet acceptance is probably the best way to describe the goal of the maintenance paradigm. Since there is very little hope that the person will improve, or indeed, leave the paradigm, the energy is driven to make the inevitable comfortable and acceptable. Even the names of the facilities that play this role in the human service system portray this goal. Some names I have encountered include:

Hill Haven Rest Home
Protestant Home for Incurables
Serenity Home
Those of the Angels

As I conclude an overview of these paradigms, it is interesting to note the declining importance given the person receiving services from the paradigm. Each paradigm, in its own way, positions the expert in charge. The recipient of services is labeled and given little say in his own situation. An awareness of this downward trend and devaluation of recipients, however, is vital in understanding interdependence.

Our human service system has established a mindset that says that those who need to receive services are not as valuable, competent, or contributing as those that do not need services. This theme suggests, then, that the person with a disability has very little to offer. Not only do they need help, but they don't contribute much in return. This cycle of deviance and devaluation of people must be acknowledged before interdependence can happen.

As we will see in the next chapter, interdependence focuses on the skills, abilities, and contribution that people with differences can offer. This shift in emphasis is critical, but it cannot happen until we are conscious of the status quo that promotes deficits.

Before we explore interdependence then, a summary of the themes common to all four paradigms is as follows:

❖ Client has the problem
❖ People are homogeneously congregated
❖ They are usually segregated
❖ They are controlled by experts
❖ Main goal is to fix, change, or maintain

Without question, a change is in the wind and a paradigm shift is imminent. The consumer lessons of the 60s, civil rights and human rights efforts of the 60s and 70s, the women's movement and ecology efforts of the 70s and 80s, and the South African and Eastern Europe changes of the 90s are creating a powerful basis for this is paradigm shift. Things must change, and interdependence can be a methodology to make the changes in human services happen.

As we shift now to explore a new paradigm, it is fitting to close this chapter with a powerful quote from John Gaventa (1989). As director of the Highlander Center in Tennessee, John and his colleagues have been working tirelessly for social change and one method for change is through participatory research. This approach positions the subjects of the research in control of the process and analysis. This idea indeed, has clear and vital implications for interdependence.

Fundamental questions must be raised about what knowledge is produced, by whom, for whose interests and towards what ends. Such arguments begin to demand the creation of a new paradigm and organization of science - one that is not only for the people, but is created with them and by them as well.

John Gaventa

3

Interdependent Paradigm

What we do with our lives
individually is not what
determines whether we are
a success or not;
what determines whether we
are a success is how we
affect the lives of others.

A. Schweitzer

3

Interdependent Paradigm

THE MEANING OF THE WORD

Interdependence is not a new concept. It is often applied to geopolitical issues. Quite simply, it is a term that implies an interconnection, or an interrelationship between two entities. In geopolitical terms, interdependence suggests a connection or partnership between countries in an effort to maximize potential of both countries. A good example of interdependence was the liasonship of allied countries in support of Kuwait against Iraq during the Gulf War. The allies forged an interdependence to promote an economic and social stabilization of all the countries involved. As I was preparing this manuscript, I researched the term *interdependence* at the University of Pittsburgh Hillman Library. I found some 40 entries in the computer that responded to the describer, *interdependence*. As I reviewed these entries, I found that all but one related to economic or political affairs. The one that was not political, focused on a psychiatric concern. Suffice it to say that interdependence has not been understood or embraced by human services.

Of course, the term has been used in relationship to human endeavor. Ghandi, and others who followed in his philosophy, such as Martin Luther King, Jr., have used the term *interde-*

pendence to describe the linkage of people to people. To them, interdependence is the destiny of freedom. King summarized this when he said:

> *In a new sense all life is interrelated. All persons are caught in an inescapable network of mutuality, tied to a single garment of destiny. Whatever affects one directly affects all indirectly. I can never be what I ought to be, and you can never be what you ought to be until I am what I ought to be. This is the interrelated structure of reality.*

King, Ghandi, and others suggest that our futures are interrelated, that none of us are free if any of us are vulnerable and that interdependence is a natural course for protection.

More recently, Steven Covey (1989), writes about interdependence in *The 7 Habits of Highly Effective People*. He introduces a maturity continuum, and suggests that dependence is the paradigm of you; independence is the paradigm of I; and interdependence is the paradigm of we. He states:

> *Independent thinking alone is not suited to interdependent reality. Independent people who do not have the maturity to think and act interdependently may be good individual producers, but they won't be good leaders or team players. They're not coming from the paradigm of interdependence necessary to succeed in marriage, family, or organizational reality. Life is, by nature, highly interdependent. To try to achieve maximum effectiveness through independence is like trying to play tennis with a golf club - the tool is not suited to the reality.*

I was excited to find Covey's perspective on interdependence. Although he uses it as a personal tool, the reference to it, and the viability he develops, offers a real synergy for my organizational application.

Covey continues his review of personal interdependence by stating:

> *Interdependence is a choice only independent people can make. Dependent people cannot choose to become interdependent. They don't have the character to do it; they don't own enough of themselves...As you become truly independent, you have the foundation for effective interdependence.*

This is an interesting perspective when you apply it to rehabilitation. Usually medically-oriented rehabilitation is focused toward independence as an end point or final goal. In Covey's analysis, however, to be independent is to be only half way there. There is much more to life and success than just independence. In fact, in a more pure analysis independence is an autonomous concept — that people are capable of taking care of themselves and being on their own. Yet this very thrust can lead down a lonely road. Clearly, people need people, and independence as a goal can push people to an autonomy that can be disconnecting. Rehabilitation has to shift beyond the goal of independence.

I feel Covey's analysis of interdependence, ushers in a strong preface for my application for interdependence to human services. Although some of my thoughts apply it differently, the basic foundation of relationships and interrelationships are consistent. My use of the term is multifaceted and paradigmatic in nature.

The interdependent paradigm is, indeed, a major shift from the four previously-discussed paradigms. Perhaps the best way to show the stark differences is to compare them side by side:

INTERDEPENDENCE	MEDICAL/EDUCATIONAL REHABILITATION
Focuses on capacities	Focuses on deficits
Stresses relationships	Stresses congregation
Driven by consumer	Driven by expert
Promotes micro/macro	Promotes fix or change

Interdependence is about relationships that lead to a mutual acceptance and respect. Although it recognizes that all people have differences, as a paradigm, it promotes an acceptance and empowerment for all. It suggests a fabric effect, where diverse people come together in a synergistic way to create an upward effect for all.

Using the same type of analysis as with the other paradigms, we can inspect the interdependent paradigm as it relates to people with disabilities in the following manner:

INTERDEPENDENT PARADIGM

The Problem	Limited or nonexistent service
Core of Problem	In the system
Actions of paradigm	Create supports and empower
Power Persons	The consumer
Goal of Paradigm	Develop relationship

This review offers a fundamentally different perspective on disability. Although the challenge is the same, the approach is radically different. I liken the fundamental difference portrayed by interdependent paradigm to a hologram. Although the picture a hologram portrays is the same when viewed from different angles, the color, depth, and "reality" of the picture can look very different. Same is true with the interdependent paradigm. When applying it to the same problem analyzed by the medical paradigm, the outlook is vastly different. Colors, depth, and implied actions can all be different when analyzed through the lens of interdependence. Let's now shift to examine each of these categories separately.

THE PROBLEM

In a refreshing way, the interdependent paradigm defines the problem of disability not from what is wrong with the person, but from the context of limited supports to allow the person with a disability the opportunity to participate. That is, rather than look at deficits or limitations that people have, it repositions the problem to be a deficit in the system by not having appropriate supports for full participation for all. It suggests a narrowness of supports, rather than an incapability of certain people to participate.

In this paradigm, it is not people who are problems, but the limited viewpoints of others. To this extent, the major problem experienced in an interdependent paradigm is attitudinal. An example of this perspective of the problem might be found with an organization that I spent some time with recently.

This group was concerned with opportunities that should be afforded to people with head injuries. When I first met with them, I realized that they had no persons who had survived head injury on their board. When I pointed this out, they responded that most survivors of head injuries have cognitive deficits that make their participation on the board difficult. I suggested that the problem is not that survivors of head injury have cognitive difficulties, but that the board has not been adjusted to function in such a way that survivors could really participate.

In this example, the organization in question was operating out of a quasi-medical paradigm. That is, if they found a survivor who was "fixed," they could then have consumer representation on their board. The real issue here, however, is not a "fixed" survivor, but a "fixed" board. The interdependent paradigm acknowledges that some survivors of head injuries do have some difficulties with cognition. With changes and adjustments made in the system, people with cognitive challenges should still be incorporated into that system and have appropriate supports.

Rather than change people to fit their board, the interdependent solution is to adjust the way the board does business to insure that even those with memory, or organizational challenges could be included. They could have used audio tapes for recording progress; perhaps a timer to assure that the board stays on task; the dates, time and place of meetings to correspond with people's strengths to participate; a mentor system so that all members become sensitized.

This fundamental shift in problem perception is critical to a comprehension of interdependence. With disability is the problem of unemployment because people have disabilities, or because we don't have adequate job supports? Is the problem of homelessness or substandard housing because people have disabilities, or because we don't have an adequate, accessible, affordable housing? Is the problem of transportation because people with disabilities can't get on buses or because we don't have accessible public transportation? These are all powerful and logical questions; and they demand viable answers.

This notion of the real problem in disability issues has further personal implications. As we discussed in the section of role expectation, if people with disabilities are constantly positioned as the problem, soon all of us begin to believe they are the problem. People with disabilities begin to see themselves as the problem and the non-disabled start to look for them to be the problem. Then the cycle of dependency and devaluation intensifies.

Over the years, many of us have followed the public career of Jesse Jackson. For those who have, the picture of Jesse Jackson meeting with poor children, having them chant, "I am somebody," "I am good," is etched in our minds. This effort is not a public relations ploy, but a paradigm shift around those who are perceived to be the problem. Just about daily, these children are told, directly or indirectly, that they are problems; that they are no good. Then here comes Jesse Jackson, a minority who has emerged as a leader and hero, telling them that they are somebody, and that they are good. This is a paradigm shift in defining the problem.

CORE OF THE PROBLEM

Every thinker puts some portion of an apparently stable world in peril.

J. Dewey

If the problem of the interdependent paradigm rests with limited supports and attitudinal barriers, then the root of the problem is found in the system. Simply stated, if we can change and extend the system to accept and welcome people with disabilities, then these people will have real opportunities.

Our current medically driven system attempts to create artificial answers through segregative programs that are offered to people with disabilities. For example, group homes do not necessarily solve the problems of community living faced by people with disabilities who live within them. In fact, at times they can further isolate and position the resident as odd to the community at large. Just creating a program or a setting does not necessarily lead way to people becoming connected and accepted in the community.

An interdependent approach sees the core of the challenge resting both in the human service system and the community at large. To this extent, the problem of community living is not answered by group homes, but inclusive opportunities for people to live in communities of their choice, with people of their choice. The problem of limited employment is not solved by segregated special workshops, but through viable jobs that have been restructured and are supported in a way that lead to valued work roles.

It is important to understand this dual challenge. On one side, we have the human service system that has emerged with its programs and services. This is that ever-growing constellation of human service agencies, all vying to make life better for their client. Today in any given community, we have the laundry list of either diagnostic, or topical groups that are devoted to a particular population or cause.

On the other hand, we have the community at large. This is both the formal and informal structure of society. This includes the guy next door, the mayor of your town, the governor of your state and the basic person on the street.

Most of these community people don't really acknowledge the "disability movement" or the struggles faced by people who are disenfranchised. Some may have a sensitivity, but, by and large, they feel that the human service system or the government will take care of the problem. To them, there is no real problem.

As we examine the community as one of the aspects of the challenge within an interdependent paradigm, it is important to clarify that the community alone is not necessarily malicious about this posture. In fact, given the historic propensity of the expert paradigms to cluster people, the community at large has not had adequate opportunity to really know people with disabilities. That is, because the historic tendency of the human service system is to segregate and congregate people with disabilities, the community has not had a viable opportunity to know or draw conclusions about these folks. Those who have, indeed, are influenced by the message of the medical paradigm about deficits and problems. They have probably assumed some of the roles that were articulated previously in this text. Thus, as we use the interdependent paradigm to move forward, we need to test out the real feelings of the community for people with disabilities. Nothing should be taken for granted.

To me, the far more challenging aspect of the core of the problem, rests with the human service system. As we explored in Chapter 2, agents of all four paradigms lock in hard as experts. In many ways, the key to the solution is getting agents of these paradigms to recognize the unfortunate iatrogenic role they can play. It is hard enough for agents of the paradigm to see the nature of the interdependence argument, let alone acknowledge that they are indeed part of the problem.

ACTION OF THE PARADIGM

The actions of the interdependent paradigm are all designed to promote and empower the distantiated person to take more charge of their life. They focus on capacities and keep the focal person of the paradigm clearly in the center of the plan. Some basic actions are:

1. Allow the Consumer to Define the Problem

The first phase of interdependence is to have people define their own problems. In all the paradigms previously described, the experts define the problem. Often, they do so by using elaborate tests or assessments that focus on the deficits or shortcomings of the person with a disability.

Interdependence, however, suggests that the consumers must have the right and privilege to determine their own situation. Most often, this is done by being heard. Regardless of situation, they are quite capable of recognizing their own reality. Even if the expert does not agree with their assessment, it seems that common sense should dictate this is where the process starts. Perception is reality, and if the person perceives his problems a certain way, then this is their reality.

This concept is probably best understood when we look at the philosophy that undergirds the Highlander Center in Tennessee. This folk school was founded in 1932 by Myles Horton as a place where oppressed people could take stock of their situation and make some decisions about what they needed to do for their cause. Horton learned early in his career, that you can't teach people things that they do not know. Rather, you must allow people to learn the things they already know.

The Center, which birthed the labor movement of the 30s and 40s, as well as the civil rights movement of the 50s and 60s, never positioned itself as a place that could teach people new things. Instead, Highlander served to allow people a chance to come together to define their own problems, then develop solutions to these problems. Horton and his staff were mere catalysts to the process, not the experts who had assessed the situation and then understood the perfect remedy.

The first big task of interdependence is thinking and understanding each other -- that means talking together.

R. Bellah

In his book, *The Long Haul*, Horton (1990), describes the development of Highlander and the educational theories of empowerment. He states:

> It is very important that you understand the difference between your perceptions of their problems, and their perceptions of the problem. You shouldn't be trying to discover your perception of their perception. You must find a way to determine what their perception is.

This challenge of letting people call their own problems is a difficult one. First, we are so conditioned to want to predict, analyze, or know what is wrong with people that to do anything else seems unnatural. For most of us out of the medical paradigm, this is not just a tendency, but an instinct. And, as we know, instincts and habits are very hard to overcome.

Second, people with disabilities are equally used to others telling them their problems, so they naturally yield to the expert. This conditioned aspect of learned helplessness can also become habitual. It's all so natural, that to do anything else seems awkward.

In an illuminating article, *Working with Women of Color: An Empowerment Perspective*, Lorraine Gutierrez (1989) states:

> Accepting the client's definition of the problem is an important element of an empowering intervention. By accepting the client's definition, the (social) worker is communicating that the client is capable of identifying and understanding the situation. This technique also places the client in a position of power and control over the helping relationship, and it does not preclude bringing up new issues for exploration, such as the connection between personal and community problem.

Gutierrez and Horton both understood the vital elements of empowerment and self direction. People must have the opportunity to call their shots, and the interdependent paradigm is predicated on this notion.

In thinking about empowerment, we must emphasize the importance of self-esteem. For persons to seize power, lack of personal faculties to deal with responsibilities can be problematic. People must have equal opportunity to explore the dimensions of their esteem and capacities. Many organized efforts toward empowerment are convinced that self-esteem issues are vital and closely related to self-direction.

Recently, a friend and colleague on disability issues, Gerry Bush, sent me the final report of the California Task Force to promote Self-Esteem and Personal and Social Responsibility, titled *Toward a State of Esteem* (1990). Gerry and I have had many discussions on the concept of interdependence. He felt the report would be helpful to my thesis. Indeed he was right. The California study recognizes the critical dimension of self-esteem in addressing any aspect of devaluation. They suggest that the following themes are vital to self-esteem and self-direction.

I. Appreciating Our Worth and Importance
   ❖ Accepting ourselves
   ❖ Setting realistic expectations
   ❖ Forgiving ourselves and others
   ❖ Taking risks
   ❖ Trusting ourselves and others
   ❖ Expressing our feelings
   ❖ Appreciating our creativity
   ❖ Appreciating our spiritual being
   ❖ Appreciating our minds
   ❖ Appreciating our bodies

II. Appreciating the Worth and Importance of Others
   ❖ Affirming each person's unique worth
   ❖ Giving personal attention
   ❖ Demonstrating respect, acceptance, and support
   ❖ Setting realistic expectations
   ❖ Providing a sensible structure
   ❖ Forgiving others
   ❖ Taking risks
   ❖ Appreciating the benefits of a multicultural society
   ❖ Accepting emotional expressions
   ❖ Negotiating rather than being abusive

III. Affirming Accountability for Ourselves
   ❖ Taking responsibility for our own decisions and actions
   ❖ Being a person of integrity
   ❖ Understanding and affirming our values
   ❖ Attending to our physical health
   ❖ Taking responsibility for our actions as parents

IV. Affirming our Responsibility Toward Others
   ❖ Respecting the dignity of being human
   ❖ Encouraging Interdependence, autonomy and competence
   ❖ Creating a sense of belonging
   ❖ Developing basic skills
   ❖ Providing physical support and safety
   ❖ Fostering a democratic environment
   ❖ Recognizing the balance between freedom and responsibility
   ❖ Cooperating and competing
   ❖ Serving humanity

Clearly, self-esteem is a foundation concept in interdependence. The California study (referenced in detail in the Bibliography section) offers important ideas and directions for self-esteem and self-direction. An important notion, however, is that those around the person who has been devalued must appreciate, acknowledge and accept the individual's definition of the situation. As I reflect on this challenge of interdependence these three A's are essential. Think about them again. Write them on a note card; put them above your desk. Reflect on them often.

Appreciate!

Acknowledge!

Accept!

These are the themes that all other interdependent actions flow from.

2. Focus on Capacities

Without question, another major action of the interdependent paradigm is to pay attention to capacities. So much time and energy of the other paradigms is deficit-oriented, that even a modest shift to capacities is face-slapping. Yet everyone has capacities, gifts, and things they can offer or contribute. Even the most severely challenged person you might know, has something that can be identified as positive.

As with the first action, however, our natural tendency promoted by the other paradigms is to look for what is wrong, weak, or dysfunctional with people. We literally need to retrain ourselves to look for capacities.

In their excellent book on Futures Planning, *It's Never Too Early, It's Never Too Late*, Beth Mount and Kay Zwernik (1987), discuss in detail the concept of capacities. In their process of Futures Planning, they suggest that support people need to learn how to conduct a "capacity hunt." To do this, support people should list out all the capacities common to the focal person. These can be things as obvious as skills and abilities, to things as simple as a smile, or bright eyes.

It is important to appreciate that a focus on capacities is not akin to a strength/needs list. Traditional medical paradigms use the strength/needs approach to develop individual program plans (IPP). These IPP's are the backbone of expert-driven paradigms, but usually, they end up staying focused on the needs and offer only lip-service to the notion of strengths.

Know too, that the concept of capacities is different from that of strength. Usually strength refers to the things that the person can do that are defined by the expert as important. Capacities, on the other hand, may have nothing to do with activities, skills or any other aspects that are considered important to the experts. They can be interests, preferences, attributes, or gifts. In this sense, they may not necessarily make the person more capable or autonomous. Indeed, as Beth Mount implores, the notion of capacity and the role it plays in futures planning is as important and viable as skill oriented strengths.

When I think about capacities the story that captures the point revolves around my friend, Bill. For years he was in a nursing home. Further, his challenging behavior had positioned him as a considerable problem. Few people saw any viable capacities in Bill.

As we were working to help Bill get out of the nursing home, one of our staff was taken by Bill's depth of thinking and spirituality. This capacity only surfaced when Bill felt optimistic about leaving the home, but when it did, it was powerful. Needless to say, this spiritual capacity opened all kinds of doors for Bill.

Without question, we need to remind ourselves to look and listen for the good things people bring to the table. The Interdependent paradigm demands it.

3. Importance of Relationships

The key dimension of interdependence is found in relationships. Often with the other paradigms, the most important relationships in the lives of people with disabilities are with the experts and paid staff who surround them. This can be related to the abandonment experienced that may result when a disability occurs. As old friends get replaced by social workers, case managers and attendants, natural relationships transfer to the paid experts. Then as people with disabilities are congregated, friendship vacancies are either filled by the experts (if they deem this appropriate), or with other people with disabilities.

This notion is strongly captured by Forest (1988) and her associates at The Center for Integrated Education and Community in the insightful training video titled, *With a Little Help from My Friend*. In her work, Forest has encouraged school systems in Ontario, Canada to accept and incorporate students with severe disabilities into the regular classroom. As these students enter the neighborhood schools, circles of support are constructed with the students and their peer with a disability. The results have been unbelievable.

To illustrate the importance of relationships to the students, Forest used a social networking technique. She asks the children to draw a circle and identify the people most important to them. Next, they are instructed to draw a second circle, around the first, and identify those that are important friends. Finally, they are asked to do a third circle and to identify those that touch their lives, but are lesser important.

As they see how vital their friendships are, she then illustrates how children with disabilities usually have nothing more than a team of experts and paid professionals in their lives. The differences are stark.

With the interdependent paradigm, it is essential that people with disabilities have adequate opportunities to establish a wide range of relationships. To this extent, experiences that will promote maximum exposure to non-disabled people are critical.

When I think about this point on relationships, and especially the void in opportunities for natural, freely-given exchanges for people with disabilities, I recall a situation with another friend, Bill. After his head injury, Bill experienced the typical exodus of his friendship network. Of course, extensive isolated rehabilitation in a far off city didn't help.

In any event, as our organization worked to facilitate natural relationships for Bill, he had the opportunity to connect with the next door neighbor in the apartment complex we helped him retain. Over the next few weeks, Bill and his neighbor started to share time.

One night, after they had watched the Pittsburgh Steeler football game on TV and his friend had left, Bill called me at home. After the pleasantries, he said, "What is the story with my neighbor, Frank?"

Not sure of his point, I asked what he meant. He responded, "Why does he hang with me, is he a new staff?" I said, "No." "Well, then is he a student, trying to get some credits for field work?" Bill asked. I again, said, "No." "Then he must be a Christian trying to convert me or get some grace points?" he asked in a serious tone.

I told him I wasn't sure if Frank was Christian, only that he is a neighbor and wants to be a friend.

After some silence he said, "Geeze, Al, then he must be lonelier than me!"

As I reflect on this story, I am struck by innocent humor. I am also saddened by the powerful message. Bill was so conditioned by the prevailing medical paradigm, his deficits, and a world of experts, that he could not even see how he could be attractive as a friend to Frank. In his mind, there had to be a real reason why Frank would want his company.

To achieve interdependence mandates that we understand the reasons why friendships break up after injury, or for the person with a congenital defect rarely form in the first place. Then we need to turn our attention to the ways whereby people can have the opportunity to forge new acquaintances that can mature over time.

4. Develop Supports

Since the interdependent paradigm accepts people as they are, and is not caught up in trying to change or fix people, another major action is to acknowledge and develop supports. In other words, we need to allow for the unique manifestations brought on by the disability, and to get people the supports that will help them enjoy life.

I am amazed by the tremendous pressure put on people with disabilities to do things that either they just cannot do, or if they can do them, the time and energy it takes is ridiculous. To spend countless hours teaching someone a task that may be impossible, or never achieved, could be a waste of time and money. Marc Gold (1980), in his work on *Task Analysis*, referred to a concept he called zero-based learning. By this he suggests that often the rehabilitation plans include items that have little to do with real life.

In many regards, this is seen time and time again in rehabilitation programs today. The typical scenario is to have the client assessed and then measured on his current ability to perform the task. He is rated at a certain level and then given a goal plan to achieve a target level. Then as time and energy is put into this goal the "client" is pushed further up the scale of performance.

The tragedy of this scenario however, is when the target goal is unrealistic and just plain unrelated to more important elements of life. In these cases, people are pushed to frustration or to a point where they could care less. Unfortunately, this scene happens all too often in our programs today.

I remember once visiting a program in the Midwest, a community reentry effort for people with developmental disabilities. As we were touring, I was drawn to a woman sitting at a work corral, writing her name over and over. Upon further inquiry, the tour guide told me the woman was practicing her name for when she returns to the community. I asked how long she had been attempting to master this skill, and the guide said nonchalantly, "two years." Think about this! For two years, this woman was practicing the writing of her name. *Two years!* And every minute of time she invested in this goal, was time away from people, developing relationships, and making connections. This says nothing about whether this woman was getting any better at the name-writing skill. Sure, the tour guide said she had improved from the 30th to 40th percentile in this time.

To this point, I don't mean to suggest that all skill building is unnecessary. Certainly, there are many skills that people can and should reacquire. Indeed, in Chapter 4, I look closely at the importance to build skills for success in important community roles.

Rather, I think we need to recognize that when a disability gets in the way of performing important tasks, there are two basic ways to proceed. One is to reteach the skill or task. The other is to get someone (or something) to do the task for the person.

Often the expert paradigms stress the first to the exclusion of the latter. This propensity to reteach, again is habitual to the medical/educational paradigm. In fact, at times, it cuts so deep, that things are taught that are not within the interest or experience base of the person.

I've toured rural programs and saw people with disabilities from urban environments being taught how to milk cows and tend field. This alone is not bad; the real tragedy is that the ultimate goal for these folks was to return to the urban setting after their rehabilitation was "completed."

In my experience, I have come across examples where people who have been injured, are taught things thought by the experts to be important, and pushed into a life-style that is very different from their pre-injury life. This approach is not only oppressive, but arrogant.

For staff to promote values they think are important can be a dangerous posture. This assumes that the staff's values are not only viable, but consistent with what the person may want. This may or may not be. Sometimes the values promoted are those of the family, or that of the expert, and not the person's. Further, if the person cannot perform the ascribed task, he is often positioned as a failure, or as someone who just did not try hard enough. This is madness.

When I think of support action, I think of an excellent quote pulled from an article by sociologist, Irv Zolla (1986), of Brandeis University in Waltham, Massachusetts. He states, "Independence should not be measured by the quantity of tasks one can perform by themselves, but by the quality of life one can have with supports."

We all need and use everyday supports to make our lives more enriched. This same spirit should surround the way we relate to people with disabilities.

5. System Change

A final action of interdependence is to recognize that the expert paradigms discussed have cut deep into our system. Without question, they have led to laws, customs, and activities conditioned to people with disabilities. To this extent, the interdependent paradigm suggests that broader, more sweeping actions must be promoted. These are actions that challenge the status quo and attempt to reframe the system that keeps people with disabilities harnessed and separate.

Perhaps the most successful example of interdependent systems action is the passage of the American's with Disabilities Act, (ADA), July 1990. This civil rights legislation sets the tone for a new America. It establishes a basic right for people with disabilities to be in and of our system. From access to transportation, to communications, ADA provides entry to American opportunities.

Another key systems action that is essential to interdependence is national Medicaid reform. Since 1984, Medicaid reform has been considered and debated by the U.S. Congress. As our current national Medicaid program is not only medical in nature, but institutional in design, and since most people with disabilities rely on Medicaid, many disability advocates contend that the potential for community activities will only happen when Medicaid is reformed.

Currently, most services offered through Medicaid can only be attained by entering an institution. That is, if a person with a disability needed attendant services, and was Medicaid eligible, the most common way they could access that service would be through admission to a nursing home. In most American states, they could not get this service and remain in the community. These present limitations are tremendously compromising to people with disabilities.

Again, this type of skewed program is a deep rooted manifestation of the medical paradigm that has been woven into law. The assumption is that all people with disabilities who might have quasi-medical needs must be institutionalized. It is as if they cannot understand their physical needs and should not have any control over basic supports for these needs.

Over and above the general push to reform Medicaid, some disability advocates feel that currently proposed national attendant services should not be tied to Medicaid at all. They contend that regardless of reform, Medicaid will remain medically dominated. They hold that attendant services must be separated from the medical paradigm to really allow people with disabilities to have control. Since many people with disabilities are dependent on attendant services, they must be readily available, and nonmedical in nature.

This issue of medicalization of attendant services is a strong one. In Pennsylvania, in 1985, we were able to obtain state-funded attendant services. When the program was initiated, disability advocates played a direct role in developing and overseeing the design. We were all pleased with the nature and intent of the services. The program was nonmedical and had built-in elements of consumer control.

Slowly, however, medical issues started to creep into the program design. First, it was the nursing lobby, contending that nurses should be involved in direct care. Next, physicians were involved in needing to insure that people were, indeed disabled.

If that wasn't enough, the wage and hour bureaucracy entered the picture, demanding that consumers pay the right taxes and benefits to attendants. Within four years, a unique program had drifted into a typical, medically-driven welfare program, where agencies dominated.

Interdependence demands that whenever new programs are achieved, they must remain in the spirit and integrity of consumer control. To work hard to obtain something, only to see it converted to an expert paradigm, is hardly worth the effort. This underscores the importance of advocacy.

In spite of this drifting and perversion found in system advocacy, we must continue the struggle. ADA is a viable start, and the pivotal systemic introduction of interdependence.

Medicaid reform and attendant services legislation are equally important. We need to move forward and pledge to be vigilant to the cause of supports that are relevant, consumer-controlled and dignified. Next, we need consistent regulations, and then swift enforcement. Finally, we must continue to monitor and assure that the program does not drift. The interdependent paradigm contends that we be conscious and competent in the ways of systems advocacy.

POWER PERSON

Perhaps the most dramatic manifestation of the interdependent paradigm is found in consumer control. Over and above the right to define the problem, interdependence strongly upholds that the consumer be in charge of all that affects their lives. This notion, however, is not easily appreciated, even by those who claim to actualize interdependence.

Time and time again, when I participate in workshops or lecture on interdependence, people challenge this concept. I've heard all the dissensions:

❖ "People with disabilities haven't had enough experiences"
❖ "You just don't understand head injury"
❖ "It may work for some people, but not all"
❖ "Some people just aren't ready"
❖ "Cognitive deficits don't permit it"
❖ "Control is only for those who can handle it"

Certainly this idea of consumer control is one that needs thought and review. The interdependent paradigm starts with the notion of consumer control. Much like our legal credo, "innocent until proven guilty," consumer control, in my opinion must come from the same place. I believe that people must be deemed capable to be in control of their lives, and only challenged if family, support people and advocates are convinced, beyond a shadow of a doubt that they are not.

Often, however, the expert paradigms take just the opposite approach. People are held accountable to prove to a host of doubters that they are capable. Additionally, the proof of capability is conducted in practice or experimental settings and is judged by experts, often looking for the person to "foul up." This indeed is the nature of the medical/educational paradigms. Solid proof is mandated prior to moving into the next step.

This notion of proof to move through the system is a powerful way in which people with disabilities are kept out of control. Just when the person achieves the goal, there is another step or stage of the continuum that puts the "client" right back to "go." Steve Taylor (1987), from the Center on Human Policy at Syracuse University, calls this the "continuum trap" (1987). To this point he stated:

> One end of the continuum represents the most restrictive or most segregated placements although this end is also sometimes thought of in terms of the most intensive services. The opposite end of the continuum represents the least restrictive or most integrated placements or least intensive services. The assumption is that every person with a (developmental) disability can be placed somewhere along the continuum, while those with mild disabilities will be at the least restrictive end. As people acquire additional skills, they are expected to move to less and less restrictive placements.

Along this scale, Taylor suggests that the "continuum trap" promotes a "readiness model" which is some outside perception that the person has now proven that they are ready for the next step. He warns, however, that this process continuously uproots people and keeps them in a constant state of flux.

As I reflect on Taylor's "continuum trap," I find a process that also continues an assault on one's self-esteem and capacity of self-direction. As the person moves to the next level, a new battery of experts jump in to define the problem and set the goal for completion.

There are three problematic features here. One is that the person with a disability must prove or perform their capabilities in less than real settings along the continuum. These settings are either set up as mock, practice, or role play situations. Often this "make-believe" setting creates a play-like tone that doesn't seem to be important. What follows is that the student just doesn't learn. Remember, role expectation leads to role behavior and if the expectation is play or practice, some people will behave accordingly. Quite simply, when something is not real, people will not take it seriously.

Another problem relates to the expert who is usually asked to judge capability. Typically, these are trained clinicians looking for problems. They have a skillful eye for faults. In some cases, they are driven through years of clinical practice and preparation to find one more problem to work on. In other situations, they just need to prove their worth to their system. Regardless, when the clinician is the sole judge of how the person measures up, there can be room for perversion.

A final concern is how people are measured or rated. I am always amazed by training situations that rate capabilities to typical norms. These are often found in vocational or independent living programs where a particular skill or task is analyzed using the performance of non-disabled groups.

For example, it might take a non-disabled person five minutes to brush his teeth, from start to finish. Taking this as the norm then, plans are set to teach and rate the person with a disability using these norms. Thus, when it takes a person with a disability ten minutes to do the same task, it is said that the person is functioning at the 50th percentile in teeth brushing. Interdependence contends that this is not only ridiculous, but inappropriate. It often holds people against standards that are not achievable.

Related to this final point, we also need to consider rating scales themselves. There are currently debates that rage in the area of competency measurement. Even the basic question of who is competent and incompetent is cloudy. Leading experts in ethics and competency continue to research this area. Many are contending that most standardized tests in competency have major flaws. Some are culturally biased, often irrelevant as to what they measure.

Over and above these points, most neuropsychological tests that are standard fare in rehabilitation, are predominantly deficit-oriented. That is, they usually end up measuring all that is wrong with the person. If you have never reviewed a neuropsychological report, you really ought to take the opportunity. Usually, they paint dark and depressing pictures.

I have a friend in Philadelphia who contends that rehabilitation facilities should mandate that all staff be given a neuropsychological battery. Not only would it help to sensitize staff to the rigors of this testing, but also reveal the many deficits that we all have. She told me that her boss did not accept her idea.

In most regards, the issue of control needs to be considered from a basic perspective of power. In countless situations I have seen, the issue of competence was merely a smoke screen for someone wanting to retain control over the person with a disability. Finding a deficit, and then declaring incompetence provides a convenient format for experts to maintaining control. Clinicians do it; parents do it, spouses do it, and unfortunately, our system does it. The net effect is that people are held back from the basic control over their lives for most of the things that you and I take for granted.

THE RIGHT TO RISK AND LIABILITY

These actions force a limitation to the right to risk. Yet, this whole concept of right to risk is vital to the nature of interdependence. We deny people actions that are accessible to valued people, because we are concerned about their protection. Yet in this denial, we can take away the very essence of life itself.

This issue on right to risk is important to understand. When a person is denied the right and opportunity to take chances, he is denied a vital outlet to learning. For most of us, critical learning is acquired when we take chances. Some people call this the "school of hard knocks."

On the right to risk, Wolfensberger suggests: "...it is dehumanizing to remove all danger from the lives of the... handicapped. After all, we take for granted that there is risk and danger in our lives, and the lives of our nonhandicapped children!"

More than this, the right to risk gets to the basic elements of taking charge, and being in charge of our lives. Ed Roberts, in a *60 Minutes* interview with Harry Reasoner (1989) stated, "Without risk, there is no life." If you think about it for a minute, Roberts is dead right.

There is another factor in this question of control and risk that must be considered in the equation — that is — the issue of liability. Like it or not, we live in a society that has embraced litigation. This has good and bad points. In the business of human service however, liability and fear of litigation usually means bad things related to people with disabilities; and these bad things typically play out in control.

There is no question in my mind that many programs designed for persons with disabilities in this country are control-oriented due to fear of liability. In fact, when I am asked to consult with organizations about interdependence, and how it may relate to their programs, one of my first issues on the table is that of risk and control. For many companies, especially the for-profit organizations, the window of risk and loss in promoting Interdependence is too great for them to embrace.

Although I differ with this decision, I can respect the company that chooses to sit out community integration programs. I cannot, however, respect organizations that move to conduct community integration programs, only to have them perverted with control of their participants, direct and indirect, to lessen their exposure to litigation.

Recognize that I am not berating organizations that consider exposure and liability. A company would be foolish to do anything less. I am, however, concerned about the creeping conservatism and control I see happening in programs that claim to be vested in community integration. Most of this action only leads to oppression and domination of the recipient of services.

I believe there are ways that formal services can balance this dilemma between risk and control, but they demand a real sense of creativity. They also demand that the interdependent paradigm be in place within the organization. The other paradigms just don't allow for the kind of participant control necessary to empowerment. Some actions that I have found helpful in lessening risk are:

1. Discuss the Issue

The right to risk is an issue that needs to be discussed and reviewed by all involved.

Key aspects of risk, and how the program or supports address risky situations should be covered. These discussions should be regular and immediate and include all the players. That is, support persons and the person with a disability should hold discussions as close to the risky event as possible.

This factor of timing is a key dimension where the expert paradigms can fall short. Usually the expert paradigms follow a 9-to-5 work schedule. Paradoxically, risky events and situations often occur on week nights and weekends. Thus, the experts are not always available for an immediate discussion. If they are, it is sometimes through a beeper or as an "intrusion" to the expert.

2. Document the Disclaimer

After thorough review of the right to risk, a disclaimer should be developed, discussed, and signed by all parties. Although such documents are inadmissible in court, they do reflect the importance and seriousness of right to risk. These disclaimers should be reviewed and updated on a regular basis. They should be specific and tied to tangible, concrete situations.

Along with participants, family members, advocates, and funding representatives should all review and sign off on the disclaimer. If nothing else, they can serve as a vehicle to raise consciousness

3. Establish Patterns of Support

Perhaps the best approach in right to risk is found through adequate support patterns. In this area, the program needs to be detailed in support, but not overbearing. These patterns of supports must also be relevant and related to the lifestyle and interest of the person with a disability.

Again, the expert paradigms have difficulty with patterns of support. Typically organization provide supports in classic shifts, much like hospitals. These shifts make things relatively neat and tidy for the organization, but can fall short to schedules needed for individuals.

Many programs under-support, or over-support people based upon shifts, and not participant needs. An open-ended support system, not bound by shifts, job descriptions, and union issues, I believe, can greatly reduce the window of risk.

GOAL OF PARADIGM

Given this overview, the goal of interdependence is wrapped around a number of vital concepts. These are:

Acceptance

This means we accept people as they are, and as they want to be. This doesn't mean that we lose sight of the importance of encouragement to grow and improve. Indeed, growth is important for us all. It's that we accept people's perspective of their own situation and allow them the space and nourishment to grow "their" way.

Relationships

People want and should have access to all types of relationships, not just with family, professionals/ experts, and other people with disabilities. In fact, when you think about it, the really instructive relationships we may have had are ones with diverse people.

Opportunities

Although this concept shows up in all the expert paradigm rhetoric, opportunity is a critical goal for interdependence. People need to have chances before they can grow. In many regards, the barrier to opportunities is found in cultural and societal injustice. To this extent, then, interdependence must also look toward our macro-system for change.

And so, interdependence has simple goals. Simple, in that it identifies things we all want. Yet, the reasons and boundaries that have prevented various disenfranchised groups from attaining these simple things are complex, historical, and paradigmatically driven. They are etched in the *status quo* way things have always been done. They demand that we think, yet as John Dewey said, "Every thinker puts some apparently stable aspect of the word in peril." Thinking causes us to challenge neutrality. Often, as Emerson said, "To think, is to differ."

Indeed, we can't be neutral with interdependence. It is a paradigm that will not allow it. Either persons have opportunities, relationships, and acceptance, or they do not. Either people have control of their lives or they do not. Either people are free to make decisions, or they are not.

In his book, *The Long Haul*, Myles Horton (1990) talked about neutrality. He said:

> *I do not believe in neutrality. Neutrality is just another word for accepting the status quo as universal law. You either choose to go along with the way things are, or you reject the status quo. Then you are forced to think through what you believe. If you're going to be for something, then you have to know there's an opposite that you're against.*

To this extent, a final goal of interdependence is to get people to think, and then to act. Paulo Freire refers to this as "praxis." It is the blending of reflection and action. In another way it is also important with interdependence to think and to feel.

When we reflect with feeling, we can put ourselves in the place of the person who is disenfranchised. When we don't reflect or feel, it is easy to move on and to allow and accept things for others that we would hardly want for ourselves.

To really feel, it is imperative that we stay conscious about our actions and our work. Such consciousness is easy to talk about, but often difficult to achieve. Our hectic word and fast-paced schedule makes it easy to drift into a service zone that is restrictive and oppressive.

Jean Vanier, writes and speaks about this challenge of feeling and compassion. As innovator of the L'Arche movement (world-wide shared living between people with disabilities and non disabled) Vanier (1973) said, "Compassion is a difficult thing for us to live... So often specialized people are interested in the problem rather than the person, in the handicap rather than the person behind the handicap."

Recently, in discussing this issue of consciousness with some colleagues, we came up with a fun idea. We were preparing a paper for a national conference, and wanted to make a point about consciousness. We decided to prepare a "Consciousness Quiz," yet realize that most experts today don't always have time to reflect. To catch their attention we structured our consciousness quiz much like the health or diet quizzes you see in advertisements. We came up with the following "Consciousness Quiz" (Condeluci, Milton, Ingalls, Fenney, 1990).

CMIF CONSCIOUSNESS QUIZ

This *CMIF Consciousness Quiz* has three distinct sections. The first section is the quiz itself. This should be administered to all support people in your program. Next is the quiz interpretation sheet that "answers" the quiz questions and provides a forum for discussion.

The final section offers some group exercises to consider with your staff. Please remember that this quiz, interpretation sheet, and group exercises are offered as ways to promote a consciousness and understanding of the principle of interdependence.

CMIF CONSCIOUSNESS QUIZ
FOR COMMUNITY REHABILITATION PROGRAMS

Al Condeluci - Sandy Milton - Christopher Ingalls - Michele Feeney

Name: _____   Date: _____
Position: _____   Score: _____

INTRODUCTION AND DIRECTIONS:

The following ten questions are designed to test your consciousness. In the fast-paced, and often competitive field of head-injury rehabilitation, we sometimes lose sight of our objectives. To gauge your level of insight, please complete the test. A score sheet and overview is attached.

Each question should be answered by all staff associated with your program. Answer each question carefully and truthfully. Once completed, check against answer/interpretation sheet; score and highlight each incorrect/inaccurate response - then address the different area. Remember, this Quiz is to challenge the most ideal and highest level of thinking about people we serve. Re-administer the quiz in 30 days.

1. In considering people for our program we:

    a. only consider the person's deficits
    b. only accept people who have graduated from rehab.
    c. only accept people who are motivated
    d. consider the person's capacities

(CMIF Consciousness Quiz con't)

2. Once accepted we always start by:
    a. reviewing the person's records
    b. doing our full assessment
    c. getting to know the person, as a person
    d. talking to their parents

3. Our program functions:
    a. strictly on policy and procedure
    b. as an agent for the client
    c. on guiding principles
    d. with no structure

4. In our staffings we:
    a. let the client define his situation
    b. do a joint review of situation with client and staff
    c. determine what is best
    d. none of the above

5. People should be in the community:
    a. once they prove themselves
    b. all the time
    c. only with staff

6. Whenever we get a chance, we promote our residents via our program.

    True   False

7. You should never put your program name on your vehicles.

    True   False

8. Referring to our clients as TBI's is not always bad

    True   False

9. Having clients do work on the program grounds as therapy is not a bad practice.

    True   False

10. As a rule of thumb, we should try to hire people with head injuries to work for us.

    True   False

ACTIVITIES GUIDE FOR THE CMIF CONSCIOUSNESS QUIZ

Al Condeluci - Sandy Milton - Christopher Ingalls - Michelle Fenney

The following is an activity program that may be used in conjunction with the Consciousness Quiz to encourage staff members and administration within programs to look at their clients through a different lens. The intent is to elevate one's awareness of the ease with which Peonage, Medicalization, Segregation and *In Vivo* versus *In Vitro* performance infiltrate community integration programs.

It is our hope that following this workshop you will take these materials including the Consciousness Quiz, The Consciousness Quiz Answer Key and the Consciousness Raising Activities back to your staff to use as part of a program development exercise. We value any feedback you can provide to us regarding the impact this information had on your program. We will use this feedback to improve future presentations in the area of consciousness raising.

The following activities correspond to the first five items on the CMIF CONSCIOUSNESS QUIZ. These activities are designed to increase staff awareness in the five respective areas addressed in the first five items of the QUIZ.

ACTIVITY ONE

I. Rehabilitation planning based on outcomes reliant on strengths.

    The next time a person is admitted to your program try planning their rehabilitation program in the following manner.

    A. Through your assessment process focus on the person's cognitive, physical, functional, spiritual, family and community strengths. Do not even list "weaknesses," or "barriers." If you must list barriers, list the societal and programmatic barriers that prevent you as a clinical team from capitalizing on the individual's strengths.

(Activities Guide For the CMIF Consciousness Quiz con't)

    B. Plan the rehabilitation program based solely on this information, using the following format:

- ❖ Person's Expressed Goals
- ❖ Strengths to Reach Goal
- ❖ Plan using strengths

    C. Have someone on the team keep track of the number of times that team members gravitate toward the person's barriers.

    D. Determine whether different outcome goals were generated using this process as compared with traditional planning.

ACTIVITY TWO

A review of medical records is vital to the assessment process when a person is admitted to a program. Unfortunately the medical records can be laden with information that unwittingly "labels" the person, without adding pertinent information to assist the program. It is always interesting to find that social histories typically take up a paragraph to a page in a set of medical records that may be up to 50 pages.

II. Getting to know a person you'll spend 480 to 720 hours with.

    Organize a role-reversal one day between your staff and clients. Where appropriate, assign a specific staff member to a specific client.

    The staff member's assignment is to get to know this client as a person so well that he will be able to portray him in a role-reversal.

    1. Following the role-reversal, have a discussion with staff and clients around how this affects their perceptions of each other.

    2. Discuss how this activity changes their feelings toward each other. Did some unnecessary boundaries come down? Do you feel less pressure to be the expert?

(Activites Guide For the CMIF Consciousness Quiz con't)

ACTIVITY THREE

III. Assessing your program structure.

A wonderful exercise to test out the flexibility of your program's structure would be to present a case vignette with a controversial situation to a number of your staff (e.g., including line staff and administrators), some of your clients, and perhaps even some family members.

1. Ask each of the individuals to respond to the situation based upon an understanding of how the program operates.

2. Assess whether there is a common thread in each person's response to a situation.

3. Do the staff search for the "policy" or can they respond based upon their understanding of the program's philosophy and guiding principles?

4. Do the client's and families respond in a similar manner to the staff suggestive of a clear set of institutional guiding principles?

ACTIVITY FOUR

IV. Programs Approach to Client Staffings.

A very simple exercise that many programs still do not bother with: The next time you staff a client, have them lead the discussion of the staffing using the following outline:

1. What are the goals that you would like to meet while you are in this program?

2. How would you describe your progress to date in working toward those goals?

3. What do you need from the program to continue progress toward meeting those goals?

(Activites Guide For the CMIF Consciousness Quiz con't)

ACTIVITY FIVE

5. Community-based versus program-based community integration.

   Five years ago a fascinating study was published in a European Journal by a Dutch neuropsychologist. In this study, they were trying to identify the most accurate predictors of a head-injured individual's driving ability. The predictors included an array of neuropsychological tests, a driving simulator, knowledge tests regarding driver safety and on-the-road evaluation. Lo and behold, the best predictor of driving ability was "driving on the road!"

   A. To track how community-based your program is, simply track number of hours that a given group of clients spend in the community with licensed therapy, versus the number of hours in a therapy room.

   B. Challenge your therapists to change the ratio so that less than ten percent of the therapy time is spent in a therapy room and discuss the effects this change had on the therapist and on the client.

CMIF CONSCIOUSNESS QUIZ
FOR COMMUNITY REHABILITATION PROGRAMS

Answer/Interpretation Sheet

Each item on this quiz can be related to empowerment, valorization or interdependence issues. This answer sheet overviews each item.

(Answer/Interpretation Sheet for CMIF Consciousness Quiz con't)

1. In considering people for our program we:

   a. only consider the person's deficits
   b. only accept people who have graduated from rehab
   c. only accept people who are motivated
   d. consider the person's capacities

Too many community programs revolve around deficits. The more we continue to see people through our interpretation of their problems, the longer they will remain disempowered, devalued, and caught in the "sick role". Conscious community programs focus on capacities by using a personal futures planning approach. Everyone has deficits and capacities. Your challenge is to find and build upon people's capacities.

2. Once accepted we always start by:
   a. reviewing the person's records
   b. doing our full assessment
   c. getting to know the person, as a person
   d. talking to their parents

It is typical to initiate any new admission through a review of the records. Usually, these records are riddled with deficits and problems that the person presents. The correct approach is to set aside the records until you get to know the person as a person. Remember, however, that most people see themselves out of the lens of medicalization. They will tell you the medical line - try to look beyond this.

3. Our program functions:
   a. strictly on policy and procedure
   b. as an agent for the client
   c. on guiding principles
   d. with no structure

Any viable system, no matter the agenda, must have some structure. The real trick for community programs is to lessen (or hold down) unnecessary policies and procedures. All they do is promote bureaucracy. One way to have "informal structure" is to consider guiding principles. This offers a framework, but still allows for creative and flexible solutions.

(Answer/Interpretation Sheet for CMIF Consciousness Quiz con't)

4. In our staffings we:
   a. **let the client define their situation**
   b. do a joint review of situation with client and staff
   c. determine what is best
   d. none of the above

One of the key elements of empowerment is to let people define their own problems. Most programs don't do this, or if they do, have token consumer representation. A community "staffing" should consist of individuals defining their problems and support people making commitments to help out in the process.

5. People should be in the community:
   a. once they prove themselves
   b. **all the time**
   c. only with staff

This is a vexing issue. Many programs feel that the "client" must prove they are ready by performing in laboratory experiences. We need to remember that the magic of success in any situation is related more to the type and amount of support than to where it is rendered. We should strive to do everything in the community. Don't look for magic solutions here - figure it out on your own.

6. Whenever we get a chance, we promote our residents via our program.
   True   **False**

We must avoid "using" the people in our programs as marketing objects. These ploys only perpetuate the stigma or sick role, both which get in the way of interdependence. In fact, if we do our job and help people connect in the community, we won't need to advertise at all. People will find out about us.

7. You should never put your program name on vehicles.
   True   False

(Answer/Interpretation Sheet for CMIF Consciousness Quiz con't)

Your name or logo are traps that can stigmatize or devalue the persons you serve. When people are driven around in highly identified vehicles, they become imaged, in the spotlight, and devalued. The real task is to fit in - not to stick out!

8. Referring to our clients as TBI's is not always bad.
   True   **False**

It is always stigmatic to label. To categorize and then pro-promote people from the point of that label is dehumanizing and devaluing. We should never, in talk or writings, refer to people as TBI's. We deal with people, who happen to have an injury. In fact, the injury may be very incidental at all. This is not to say that people may not have some differences. Indeed, we all have differences. Labels are nothing more than a convenience for staff.

9. Having clients do work on the program grounds as therapy is not a bad practice.
   True   **False**

It is a bad practice, because it creates an image that this is all "they" can do and can lead to peonage. If things must be found for people to do, look to the community for options.

10. As a rule of thumb, we should try to hire people with head injuries to work for us.
    True   **False**

No we should not, at least as a rule of thumb. People with disabilities can do a myriad of things and should not all be guided toward "helping and human services". Of course, for some people with this bent, fine. In fact, the sensitivity and awareness that "peers" bring to the workforce can be great. But this should not happen as a rule of thumb.

To see how you rated please see the CMIF Consciousness Quiz Scoring Guide.

CMIF CONSCIOUSNESS QUIZ
Scoring Guide

Each correct question is worth 10 points.

100%   Excellent -- keep it up and spread the word

80-90%   Good Effort -- develop a quality circle around
                  your differences and make the move.

60-70%   Average -- Come on guys, push forward.

40-50%   Below Average -- All is not lost. Stop now and
                  have a consciousness retreat. Figure out what
                  you need to do.

30% or below Pitiful - Why do community work at all?

The real value of consciousness-raising is to bring people back to a zone of compassion. In this effort reflection leads to feelings that equate many situations. Consider these thoughts on compassion. They come from a book of meditations, designed for reflection (Hawson, 1974). Put them in the context of your life and your work.

❖   We reach a point when we become satiated with ourselves and when our life demands that we turn outward toward other human life. When we cease being the passive vessel and ourselves become the living spring.

❖   Human beings become human beings only when they have learned to feel with others, for this is the meaning of compassion. It is the crown of consciousness making the king among men, but it is a crown which any commoner may left to his own head. That crown (does not) signify conquest or power over others, but conquest and power over the self, than which there is no other real power or glory.

❖ The degree to which one is sensitive to other people's suffering, to other men's humanity, is the index of one's own humanity. It is the root not only for social living but also of the study of humanities. The vital presupposition of the philosopher's questions about man is his care for man.

Over the years, I have talked with many administrators and officials who are far removed from people with disabilities, yet they have unbelievable control over what may or may not happen in their lives. Often, these administrators have abstract, and paradigmatically skewed perspectives of who these people are. They might be perceived as numbers, or labels, or merely another of an endless cascade of clients. Yet, when personal introductions or relationships occur, magic can happen. I believe this magic is related to consciousness, feelings, and compassion.

I can remember a welfare official who visited our center with a real notion that the funding for our supports was excessive, and perhaps, unwarranted. As part of his visit, we stopped to see an individual we were supporting. Clearly uncomfortable when we entered his apartment, this official noticed a photo of some children on the coffee table and assumed they were sisters of Tim, the man we were visiting. When asked, Tim clarified that they were his daughters, and the official was amazed. I am sure he had no image of people with disabilities having children.

The real point to this story, however, related to the official's own life. He too, had daughters the same age. As he looked and talked with Tim, I could see him really feeling what it might be like to father his own daughters if he had a disability. He felt, and then could see the similarity and the simplicity of what Tim wanted in his life. They wanted the same things.

To encourage opportunities for administrators in the bureaucracy and people with disabilities to come together, the Commonwealth Institute of Pennsylvania has sponsored a series of "partnership projects." These gatherings featured a weekend retreat of Health and Welfare officials with members of the disability group "Speaking for Ourselves." According to Thomas Neuville, former director of the Commonwealth Institute, the level of understanding, compassion and commonalty of need was amazing after both groups let go of their anxieties. Once people open to each other, real progress can occur.

*Power is not only
what you have, but
what your enemy
believes you have.*

S. Alinsky

EMPOWERMENT AND INTERDEPENDENCE

If interdependence could be defined within a concept, it would be empowerment. To empower is to allow people to take charge of their situation. The word *empower*, in reality, implies taking control, or allowing people to control their own situation. Lorraine Gutierrez (1990) defined empowerment as "a process of increasing personal, interpersonal, or political power so that individuals can take action to improve their life situation." This definition suggests three key dimensions to empowerment: personal, interpersonal, and political.

In human services, and especially in rehabilitation, the intent has always been to prepare, or teach people to get back in control of their situation. Over the years, however, people with disabilities have felt that they have not been given the power. This is not all the fault of rehabilitation.

In fact, it appears that leading commentators on rehabilitation in America recognize the importance and place of empowerment. Recently, in the Archives of Physical Medicine and Rehabilitation, John Banja (1990) suggested that, "Rehabilitation is a holistic and integrated program of medical, physical, psychosocial, and vocational interventions that empowers a disabled person to achieve a personally fulfilling, socially meaningful, and functionally effective interaction with the world."

This more correct definition of rehabilitation that includes empowerment as a key component, marks a clear shift in thinking. In the same article, Banja goes on to add that, "To empower in rehabilitation, however, is to energize and catalyze a rehabilitation consumer's capacity for life, as well as to maximally enable him or her to ambulate, communicate, process information and so on."

This is a critical contention. It puts empowerment right up there with the physical, cognitive and communicative tasks. If Banja is reading the tea leaves right, and I believe he is, this article is indeed a paradigm shifting piece. It calls loud and clear in the field of physical medicine and rehabilitation, the very bastions of the field, that change is necessary, and that the profession must get ready for Interdependence.

To me, the frustrations of people with disabilities feeling that they are not given power and control of their situation, however, is related as much to a lack of community reception, as it is with rehabilitationists retaining or maintaining control. That is, as long as the community at large feels that people with disabilities are not capable of contributing to community, the longer we will have a sense of disempowerment, even if rehabilitationists shift their emphasis.

This issue in and of itself, is a justification for interdependence. However, the rehabilitation and human service community are not without their blame. As communities have distanced themselves from people with disabilities, the human service workers have rushed in to fill the void. Both of these actions have happened concurrently and both continue to frustrate people with disabilities.

In exploring this concept of empowerment, a number of factors have been identified. One study (Lord & Farlow, 1990) looked at personal empowerment with 38 people who had direct experience with being oppressed and devalued. They found four important themes that were common as people from this sample took more control in their lives. These were:

1. *Motivational trigger* — the participants all had some event or person in their life that caused them to take the first steps toward control.
2. *Alteration in environment* — most study participants had a change in venue that spurred them on.
3. *Consciousness of capacities* — As people felt more empowered, their awareness of their own capacities grew.
4. *Community involvement* — Finally, most participants mentioned that by participating in community activities they felt more empowered.

Other notions or empowerment stress the importance of linking the process of control with grounded realities our lives and community. To do this, we must find and acknowledge our common ground and values. One theorist (Bellah et. al., 1985), suggests that we need local initiatives that will be a pre-course to empowerment. These initiatives must stress common reflection and acknowledgment of what we want and need in our communities.

In looking at empowerment and its relationship to democracy, three actions are used to promote a definition (Oldendorf, 1987). These are:

1. Believing that people can be effective in addressing injustice and oppression in their lives;
2. Asking questions about the differences between democratic class and the realities of society; and
3. Acting to change society based on universal principles of benefit to all.

This definition is uplifting because it suggests a belief in people, a reflection on right and wrong and finally a willingness to act to make things better.

When I think about empowerment, I am drawn to look at other movements. History is riddled with situations where devalued groups have moved to seize, or gain power. It is prudent for us to explore common aspects of these movements.

Essentially empowerment is an internal and external voyage. On the internal side, devalued people need to explore and consider the issues of self-esteem. The better one feels about oneself and one's situation, the easier it is to take control.

This area of self-esteem cannot be emphasized enough. The prevailing medical/expert paradigms have been effective in keeping people with disabilities in inferior roles. In all honesty, with this reality, it is very difficult for wounded people to jump right up and seize control. Indeed, in situations where this has occurred, the movement has not been as successful as it could have been.

Certainly the issue of self-esteem has been explored by many people in many ways. My intention here is to acknowledge its importance and to urge its consideration in practice. My sense, however, is that the quickest way to self-esteem is to focus on capacities, give people control, and support them in their efforts.

On the external side, empowerment does have some tenets that apply for interdependence. As I have studied other movements of empowerment the key themes I have discovered are:

Sensitivity and Awareness

People who have been oppressed need to come together to acknowledge their situations, share common stories, and gain strength in numbers. Just comparing situations, learning that you are not alone, can be vitally therapeutic.

In most movements for equality, the consolidation between colleagues in the struggle is well-documented. In the early stages of the civil rights cause, the churches served as the common bond. Sundays became vital days to regroup, hear sermons relevant to the cause, and "fuel up" for the challenges ahead. It is no quirk, that most of the early leaders in civil rights were men of the cloth such as Ralph Abernathy, Martin Luther King and Fred Shuttlesworth.

Along with church, other settings, most notably the Highlander School in Tennessee, served as a critical incubator for the emerging civil rights movement of the 1950s. This rural educational retreat hosted most early civil rights leaders, allowing them the space and freedom to sort out their own passage. Indeed, Rosa Parks spent time at Highlander prior to her historic sit-in.

The bond for awareness and sensitivity during the early stages of the women's movement was found in support groups and organizations such as the National Organization of Women (NOW). This national linkage, complete with newsletter, phone network and local support groups helped keep members of the movement connected.

Finding the Targets

When frustrations are aired, they lead to the next logical question ... who does this to us? All devalued groups have targets who keep them oppressed. Some have malicious intent, others are more innocent. The point is, there is always a root cause for oppression. It is my contention that a key target for empowerment of people with disabilities is the expert paradigms previously discussed.

This notion of the target is one not to be taken lightly. Any issues of empowerment are complex ones. Finding specific points of oppression are not always easy. Allies and enemies can drift and change. Often it is easy to identify the "system" as the problem, but in any strategy development this is much to vague.

Similarly, groups advocating change need to recognize that, at times, they can be their own worst enemy. To this extent they can be the target.

In October 1989, at Galveston Texas, a national gathering of people who had survived head injuries was held. Called "Operation Empowerment" this forum followed the three external steps of empowerment: sensitivity and awareness, finding targets, and developing strategies. In the discussion about targets, many people testified that they keep themselves disempowered by believing the deficit predictions they were told by rehabilitation experts.

Strategies for Change

In empowerment, two things must change. One is the perspective of the devalued groups. Hopefully this change is toward a greater self-esteem. The other change is with the targets who have created the oppression in the first place. More of the strategies for change are articulated in other parts of this book, but it is important to note that the strategies are both internal and external. That is, in looking at power, people need gauge what must change within them, and then what must occur outside. I see these internal changes being consistent with getting a better grasp of roles and how to be more competent within these roles. Externally, organized efforts must be employed to change attitudes and systems that oppress.

Consequently, with interdependence, this process of empowerment plays out in three major arenas. These are:

1. Inside the person – to empower oneself
2. Human service system/family
3. Community at large

Before overviewing these three arenas and actions, it is important to spend a bit more time on this concept of empowerment. Know that the term *empowerment* is a hot one today. You hear it often and in the strangest of circles. Indeed, as I mentioned earlier in this text, I have visited rehabilitation programs that were anxious to show me their "empowerment programs," as if empowerment can be packaged.

For me, empowerment is the feeling one has when one is free to exercise options in solving problems. These feelings are private and differ from person to person. To be in power also mandates a responsibility and a seriousness. When a person is free to take control, he is thought to be empowered.

One theory (Keiffer, 1984), suggests there are four major stages associated with empowerment. These are:

1. *Entry* – the mutual action to take change.
2. *Advancement* – the process of moving forward in ones control
3. *Incorporation* – taking one's emerging power on an inward perspective.
4. *Commitment* – Being able to transfer one's power to commitments and relationships.

In these stages, all action happens in close context with the environment.

Another unique element about empowerment is that it can ebb and flow. That is, at times, people can be in total control and at other times, be intimidated or oppressed by others. Consider the confident business man, who is totally intimidated by his medical doctor. Or the policeman who is intimidated by a judge.

In these examples, the power shifts, based on skill or control. As confident, or esteemed people move from their sphere of power to a new area, intimidation can occur. An important notion to remember is that if the person has no base of confidence or esteem, he will never get out of the empowerment gate. Often, this is the case for people with disabilities.

When looking at how empowerment is used in the human service literature, the concept usually implies or describes political power. Certainly this is important, especially in the systems advocacy area of interdependence. Empowerment is also a concept that relates to personal power as well.

In an article, *The Power of Empowerment Language*, (Rappaport, 1985), empowerment is defined to:

> *...suggests a sense of control over one's life in personality, cognition, and motivation. It expresses itself at the level of feelings, at the level of ideas about self-worth, at the level of being able to make a difference in the world around us...We all have it as a potential. It does not need to be purchased, nor is it a scarce commodity.*

This notion puts the concept of empowerment square in the personal realm. It implies that power, at times, has little to do necessarily with politics or strength. Rather, power is a relative concept that occurs with the relationship between how we are treated, and how we perceive ourselves.

EMPOWERMENT ARENAS

Personal

Given the personal aspects of the concept of empowerment, the obvious first area for action is the individual. In Chapters 1 and 2, the case was made for how people with disabilities have been devalued and disempowered. The depth and energy of this disempowerment has left intense scars.

People who have been devalued must have opportunities and experiences to make choices and to be in charge. This action can and should happen early in the process. In fact, when I visit inpatient rehabilitation settings, I am amazed at all the opportunities for control and choice of the patients that are missed. Basic decisions about meals, activities, and room set up are often overlooked, assuming that they really are not that important, or that the individuals they serve cannot make the decisions.

Facilities should employ every opportunity in their power to promote choices, control and maximizing relationship development while people are residents. Such options could be as simple as the times when therapies or activities are scheduled to more complex issues such as conjugal visits, or assignments of staff. Any of these efforts will be steps toward empowerment and interdependence.

Another personal action for empowerment is for people with disabilities to observe, or be aware of other people with disabilities who have successfully achieved. This type of peer perspective can promote a strong sense of empowerment. Simply, people feel good about their future when they see peers who have "made it."

In our day and age, people with disabilities are just emerging in a public image that is typical. In the past, people with disabilities were either seen as objects of pity, or people of tremendous courage. These stories showed only the skewed ends of reality. Today, as Hollywood and Madison Avenue become sensitive to the realities of disability, we are seeing a more realistic portrayal. This everyday exposure can only help in the process of empowerment.

Rehabilitation/Family System

The obvious action at this level is for professionals and family members to let go of the power and allow the person with a disability to take control. Again, there are many excuses for why this cannot happen, and some of these excuses are valid. Nonetheless, the people around the person with a disability must bend over backwards to assure that personal powers are regained. At times, this may be awkward, or plain risky, but support people must allow the space. Empowerment can't happen without it.

Another action, one that will be explored in depth in Chapter 4, is for family and support people to turn their attention to educating and sensitizing the community. We must redirect our propensity to focus on the person with a disability, and go to work on the community. Support people play a vital role in reversing or changing the public portrayal of people with disabilities.

The Community

The third target in empowerment rests with the community at large. For years people with disabilities have been "out of sight, out of mind." Obviously, this will change. What becomes important, is the image of the change.

The community's present understanding of disability as stated earlier is through telethons, or courageous stories of outstanding people with disabilities. These are not typical, everyday pictures. New stories of commonality must be rendered. These will lead to new pictures of community. We cannot wait for Hollywood or television, however; it is up to us - now.

This community challenge must include us all: people with disabilities, professionals, families, advocates, and friends. It mandates a new script and role change for everyone. Interdependence offers this script.

Indeed, empowerment has forged a type of pedagogy that has been referred to as "education for empowerment" (Heany, 1982). One definition of education for empowerment is:

> *Education for Empowerment - liberatory education - seeks to develop a pedagogy that emphasizes mutual responsibility for learning and teaching, shared critical reflection on the social order, and collaboration in action. Liberatory programs are those that facilitate the development of independent, critical and politically aggressive makes of history.*

This whole concept of education for empowerment or liberatory education is again, exemplified by the work of Myles Horton and the Highlander Research and Education Center. Using the premise that education is action and that dynamic action is the foundation of social progress, actions of the Highlander Center have been chronicled in many works (Adams, 1975; Conti & Felling, 1986; Kennedy, 1981; Peters & Bell, 1986). Over the years Highlander has practiced a genuine sense of educational praxis for adults. That is, it has served as a place where people can reflect on what they need and know, and then to act on this knowledge.

Without question, Highlanders has been about empowerment, and according to Reed (1981) there are four principles to this process. These are:

❖ Use the learners' values and social interests to determine the purpose, character, and direction of the learning process;
❖ Use the social experience of the learners as the basic content, the raw material of the learning process, since there is no such thing as neutral knowledge;
❖ Link the learners' practice to the historical development of society; and
❖ Draw on the lessons and experiences of persons having similar social values and faced with parallel social conditions in order to improve the learners' own practice.

These four principles are vital to consider when thinking about educational services and the goal of empowerment. So often, the prevailing educational paradigm, as articulated in Chapter 2, drifts into the process and perverts the end result.

Thus, empowerment can be summarized to revolve around the following key points:

❖ Individuals define their own problems.
❖ They focus on capacities and abilities to promote confidence.
❖ They understand power structure and aspects of spheres of influence.

❧

*There is no failure
except in no longer
trying.*

E. Hubbard

CONCLUSION

So what do we make of all this? I believe it pushes us to examine some fundamental questions from a new light. Stop for a moment and ponder these points.

ARE WE RESPONSIBLE FOR OR TO PEOPLE WE SERVE?

Medical/educational expert models, by their controlling nature, are responsible for people. They believe people have limitations that must be acknowledged and offset.

On the other hand, interdependence makes a commitment to people. This commitment does not get lost in changing objectives or control.

SHOULD PEOPLE BE IN OR OF COMMUNITIES?

Placing people from oppressive institutions, to lesser oppressive environments can achieve that "in" objective. However, can these smaller settings really help people become of their community? I believe medical/expert paradigms, cannot lead us to this agenda.

DO WE WANT CARING LITTLE COMMUNITIES, OR COMMUNITIES THAT CARE?

Interdependence is about holistic change. It recognizes that communities abdicated their responsibilities to people with disabilities. The experts from the medical/educational paradigms have rushed in to show that they can do it better. Thus, communities have lost a sense of the gifts and contributions that people with disabilities can make. Indeed, all of us, including communities, have been taught and reinforced to believe in the deficits and limitations sold by the medical/educational paradigms about people with difference.

To this extent, then, to apply interdependence mandates that we appreciate systems theory related to holism. Consider the following graphic:

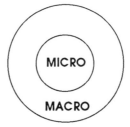

Life is a tight ecological web that links up and down the scale. Our micro worlds — our abilities, personality and character are uniquely related to our macro world — the family, friends, community and greater society. You really can't consider one without the other.

With the concept of interdependence at hand, we now need to look at ways and means to achieving the elements of this new paradigm.

4

Achieving Interdependence

*All good things which exist are
the fruits of originality.*

J.S. Mill

4

Achieving Interdependence

This concept of interdependence is a multifaceted one. The notion of connecting disenfranchised people back to their communities sounds simple. However, making it happen, is a process that must blend a number of variables. We need to recognize that, in some regards, we have to undo what has already been done.

As was mentioned previously, the historical roots of devaluation have prompted the present paradigms to become dominant. In so doing, both professionals in the disability world, as well as the community at large, have become set in their approach and ways. In some regards, we will be our own worst enemy in making interdependence happen.

FOUR FACTORS IN ACHIEVING INTERDEPENDENCE

Allowing for this, I believe there are four major factors that we must consider in achieving interdependence. Certainly, in reviewing these four factors, know that there are other dimensions that can and do relate to interdependence. I trust, however, that most dimensions are folded into the analysis of these four factors. Know too, that the key themes of the interdependent paradigm must be woven into any of these four actions. We must remember that:

1. The person with the disability be in charge of the situation. He must have as much control over his life decisions as is possible. This area should be underscored and safeguarded because it is so easy to pervert.

   I know many professionals/experts/families who say they subscribe to this principle, but find a variety of reasons to exclude the consumer from real decision making. They rationalize that the person can only offer so much, or that they have judgement or abstraction deficits that interfere with real decision making.

   Interdependence demands that people with disabilities be folded into the decision making process. In fact, if we err at all in this area, it should be on the side of people making their own decisions.

2. The person with the disability must be engaged to define the perspectives of the problems they face. They need to feel safe and secure in revealing their thoughts. Again, this is an area that can be influenced by professionals or families.

   First, many people with disabilities are conditioned to not express their perceptions, but instead to just yield to the perspectives of the professional. Indeed, there are people with disabilities I know who couch their complaints and perspective of their problems precisely in scripts designed by professionals or family members.

   Interdependence demands that support people do all they can in allowing people with disabilities to define their own situation. Extra attention must be paid to the "influence factor" of the family or professional. That is, the amount of direct and indirect influence that professionals have over people with disabilities.

Interesting enough, this "influence factor" can also play out with people outside of the medical paradigm. That is, as easily as a person with a disability can be swayed toward what professionals feel is best, so too can they be swayed by other outside people. This can have good or bad results.

We have people with disabilities being supported through our services in Pittsburgh who have chosen to associate with people I have perceived as undesirable. This puts me in a challenging spot. Do I interfere in the relationship because I think it might be problematic? Do I let it unfold without a word? If I do the latter, and things go bad, how do I answer families or funding sources?

Indeed, it is much easier and safer for a program to control what they think may be a bad influence. Yet through this control, we can oppress, disempower, and possibly intimidate. It is a hard spot.

A friend of mine, a physician with a fine program in California told me of a dilemma he recently faced. He was working with an individual with a head injury who wanted to drive. Although he demonstrated all the necessary reflexes and physical dimensions, my friend was concerned with judgement. There was nothing tangible, just a basic instinct that this man would not do well on the road. Consequently, the physician tried to dissuade him from taking the wheel.

Of course, the person in question would not buy it. He wanted to drive, and he saw the physician as interfering in his life. Certainly not being able to drive in California can be incredibly limiting.

So what was this physician to do? Where do the professional's values, instincts, and skills stop, and peoples' controls begin? These are not easy questions.

Interdependence responds with a strong endorsement of the right to risk, and the need for viable (perhaps documented) feedback on the elements associated with that risk. It promotes a shift from being responsible FOR people, to a perspective of being responsible TO people.

3. We must insure that all activities in the four areas promote the capacities of the individual. We must be cautious of our propensity to slip back into keying in on deficits. Any person we engage, regardless of the aspects that may make them appear or act differently, has some gift, capacity or contribution to make. Beth Mount and her associates call these capacities "tickets." They believe, and I agree, that we all have "tickets," and we can all use them to develop relationships. I will look more at "tickets" in the review of relationship-building.

4. We must stay focused on connecting people, not on fixing them. We have to guard that we don't analyze, predict and preset what people can do. Again,

the lure of the medical paradigm to fix and cure people of their ills is a powerful one. But interdependence is about relationships. We need to remember this and use it to guide us in the four actions to make it happen.

Keeping these "musts" in mind, let's segue to review the four actions. These are:

ACTIONS OF INTERDEPENDENCE

1. Role Competency Enhancement
2. Supplemental Supports
3. Relationship Building
4. Systems Advocacy

These four actions are things we can do in support of people with disabilities. They are highly interactive, link and relate to each other, and are all equally important. The person successful in obtaining interdependence is able to address all four, and can move in and out of any factor fluidly.

ACTION 1

Role Competency Enhancement

What is necessary, I wondered, for us to become complete human beings.

O. Sacks

When any of us are looking to do something new or different, a good first step is to enhance our skill or competency in the new challenge. For me, when I became interested in understanding computers and word processors, the logical step was to enroll in a class to learn more. When I did this, I found a fairly homogeneous groups with the same agenda. Most were my age, slightly behind the computer literacy of today's generation, but thrust into a world where we needed to know the technology. There was safety in numbers, but a real challenge to learn.

When I think of the objective of interdependence, to develop relationships, I am inclined to think the same way. What do we all need to know about relationships in order to achieve our objectives? What competencies do we need to enhance?

Now generally, the area of competency enhancement has been a mainstay of the educational paradigm, and one that has been embraced in rehabilitation for years. The usual approach, however, has been for the expert to figure out what is wrong with the person (usually through an assessment); tell them what they need to do to make these deficits better (usually through counseling); put them through the hoops to prove that they can do it (usually through a segregated, classroom-like setting); and then deem them capable or incapable.

In this approach, the onus has been on the consumer to listen passively, and then prove to the expert that he can do it. Further, this activity has usually revolved around the basic life skills, or activities of daily living (ADL). Although these actions might help someone to make a meal, write a check, or take a bath, they do not necessarily prepare a person for holding and keeping important community roles, and to learn the things one needs to know to be successful.

Thus, in competency enhancement, what I am recommending is that we all need to think, learn, and incorporate new information about roles. We must join together, in a quest to identify and itemize the important roles in our communities. Next we must analyze and dissect the key features inherent to these roles. Then we need to figure out how we can acquire the skills and competencies to successfully perform these roles. Note my focus on the word, "we."

Recognize that I think we need to back-burner the traditional things we think are important to independent living. Remember, our goal is not independence, but interdependence. This is not to imply that some (maybe all) of the life skills are not important. Sure they are, the question is how important. Further, if they are so important, why haven't they more effectively launched people with disabilities into community success?

I feel that the roles of interdependence are, in reality, more important and must be addressed first. We need to think, and try to apply strategies to enhance community success. To this extent, no one, staff, consumer, family or board, is more important, or has all the answers. Indeed, the more articulate any of us become in community roles and relationships, the more success any of us will have in life.

To this extent, in role competency enhancement, we are all teachers and students, and all have things to give and receive. Understanding community roles works for us all. There are no real experts.

Now, this is an important notion. What typically happens in rehabilitation programs is that divisions separate those who are important, and in the know, from those who are less important, and don't know. I'm sure, as you read these words, you know where you fall in the importance division. If you have some unique information, you are more apt to be powerful and in control. Thus, if you understand how muscles move as a physical therapist, you are more powerful (and important) than the person who does not know how muscles move. Similarly, if you are now successful in your ADL's, you are more powerful (and valuable) than the person who cannot perform their ADL's.

Making this the next logical step, the person who is competent in some functional area, is then usually hired or retained to teach this competence to those who are not skillful in the same area. Consequently, the action of this approach is totally downward. The script is "I know, you don't, here, let me tell you how." In this analysis, the student has very little to offer the transaction.

However, in role competence, we are all students on the same voyage. We know that the more competent we are in basic community roles, the more successful we will be in life. We have as much to gain as the person who has been ripped away from community. In a large way, the shift from ADL's to community roles, balances the equation of power, importance and value.

As I think about community role competence, the first question to confront, deals with identifying the roles critical to community success. Although there are others, I can initially offer five roles vital to the basics of community. These are:

FRIEND
NEIGHBOR
CONSUMER
CITIZEN
CONSERVER

With each of these roles we find interaction and engagement of others. They all have unique features, but also some common threads. To better understand this notion of community roles, allow me to share some personal ideas about these five roles. (Know that this is not a definitive exercise, but informal thoughts about these roles.) As you read through my thoughts, try to conjure up your own. More importantly, try to think of how you can weave this type of material into your daily work.

Friends

Friendship is a deep notion. It has been the subject of books, plays, sonnets, poems, courses, and films. A friend is something we all are, yet being a friend is something we all know we can do better. It is simple and complex, easy and hard. Friends can make us laugh and cry. What is this thing we call friendship and always take for granted?

To understand friendship and the friend role, is to ask yourself, what makes for a good friend? What do we look for in the role? What do you expect from friendships? Although we can each go through this exercise with the people we support, in my analysis here are some important things I look for from friends:

- ❖ *agreeable* – I like people as friends who are positive and agreeable. I look for people with an "up" attitude.
- ❖ *flexible* – Life is full of bends and twists. To this extent, I want to be near people who are able to bend and flex.
- ❖ *available* – Certainly, I want people for friends who are available to be connected to me. This is not to say that I want undivided attention. Only that I expect some access to those people I call friends.
- ❖ *listener* – Since friendship is predicated on communication, I want friends who can listen.
- ❖ *non-demanding* – I also want my friends to not press me too much. Certainly, I want some critiques from friends, but I get uncomfortable when there are too many demands or challenges.
- ❖ *similarity* – Although I like diversity, with friends, I seem to want some basic similarity. I am attracted to people who want the same things from life as I.

Now these are but a few of the elements of friendship that I look for. Of course, these are also the same elements I know that I need to develop if I want to attract more friends, or be a better friend. I'm sure, if you took the time now to think of friendship, you could generate a list. What is better, however, is if you would engage in this process with other people who have equal interest in friendship, your ideas and thoughts are sure to expand.

Neighbor

The notion of neighbor is crucial to community integration. As people get back to community, sooner or later they will find themselves in the neighbor role.

As I ponder the thought of good neighboring, I am reminded by people who share with me the transiency of today and society. They suggest that the idea of neighbor is a dying one, but I don't buy it. I know there are communities in America where people are less likely to consider their neighbors, but these are exceptional, and I believe, lonely places.

As Toqueville described in *Democracy in America*, one of the unique, and he felt successful aspects of American society, was the neighbor bonding that created associations. He felt that it was these associations that truly promoted democracy.

If you pause to think about your neighbor relationships, you'll probably be amazed at the importance they play in your life. People routinely call on neighbors for help, advice, a chore, a cup of sugar, and on and on. For many of us, neighbors become close and personal friends.

So, I pose to myself the same basic question: what makes for a good neighbor? What do I expect from a neighbor?

Again, you can, and should go through the exercise, and should do this with other people to enrich the process. For me, good neighbors are:

❖ *concerned about the neighborhood* – I look for people who care how our community looks and operates.
❖ *participate in community events* – I feel that good neighbors participate in the events of the community. They are interested in the quality of experiences for all.
❖ *reach out* – I want a neighbor who will be there when I need them. Somebody that cares about my welfare. This tells me that they care about the welfare of the area.
❖ *respects privacy* – Equally, I want a neighbor that respects my space and privacy.
❖ *hospitality* – Neighborhoods, indeed communities, are built on the concept of hospitality. I want my neighbor to be hospitable.

There are more, but you get the picture. Again, there are elements that we can study, discuss and practice that will make us better neighbors.

Citizen

On a broader scale, we are all citizens of our country. This moves from the informality of neighbors, to the responsibilities of citizenship.

As with friends and neighbors, the role of citizen is not without its important components. What makes a good citizen? What do I look for in assuring that citizenship?

❖ *informed* – You can't vote, or testify publicly if you are not informed. To practice good citizenship takes information.
❖ *active* – For democracy and citizenship to work, it also takes action on our part. Action to vote, to attend public meetings, to speak out.
❖ *responsibility* – Good citizens take things seriously and are responsible. When election day comes, they vote.
❖ *sensitive* – Citizenship is about society. We are a collection of people, and the welfare of each of us is vested in the welfare of all of us. Good citizens care about their neighborhood, community and country.

Consumer

The fourth important role for interdependence rests with consumerism. As consumers we find ourselves engaged in a variety of decisions about goods and services in our lives. What should we eat? Where should we eat? What products do we need? What is the best choice on these products? These, and a thousand other questions are ones we face in the community. What makes for a good consumer?

* *informed* – Again, being informed is a basic ingredient of consumerism. We need to know about products and their contents.
* *decisive* – In consumerism, we need to be good decision-makers. We must analyze our options and know how to make a smart call.
* *assertive* – There are all types of challenges in the market-place. Successful consumers are able to indicate their preferences and be able to stand their ground under competitive pressure.

Conserver

I was recently in Vancouver, British Columbia, meeting with some friends on disability issues. As I described the previous four important community roles, one of the persons I was with brought up an interesting fifth role; that of conserver. He suggested that being a constant consumer, one who is always taking from the system, might continue to perpetuate negative images. He understood the viability of consumerism, but suggested that I add the role of conserver. I agree with his point, and thank him for the addition.

In the 90s, if there is any political issue that most people would agree with, it would be conservation. We need to appreciate the elements of supply, demand, and the aspect of resources. We need to be stewards of the things we have and hold dear. We need to appreciate that when we waste, however small, that waste has a cumulative effect.

To this extent, the role of conserver has some elements that I feel are important. These are:

* *Awareness*

People who conserve are aware of the negative results of their actions, and work to make changes in their habits.

❖ *Sensitivity*

Similarly, people who conserve are sensitive to the effects of their actions.

❖ *Creativity*

Conserving demands creativity and ideas that are workable. Creativity is important.

These roles of interdependence are the stepping stones to community success. They relate to all of us, and bond us with all people who seek to belong to community. Consequently, as the interdependent paradigm looks at the micro perspective, it is competence in these, and other complimentary community roles that should garner our attention.

Enough of fixing people. We should be working to help each other culture a better community.

ACTION 2

Supplemental Supports

∽

I get by with a little help from my friends.

J. Lennon
P. McCartney

A vital dimension of interdependence is the recognition that disability, and its manifestations, can be permanent. Indeed, it is the crossing point between when a person can be fixed, and when he cannot, that creates the greatest challenge to the medical paradigm. As has been stated, the medical model is driven to make people better, the way they were before their injury or accident. When people have maxed out, the medical paradigm gets frustrated.

With interdependence, this juncture announces a shift from competency enhancement to supplemental supports. Quite simply, interdependence recognizes that no one is totally perfect and capable in every area. If a person is no longer capable in a physical area, then we modify the environment and/or bring in an attendant. If a person has incurred changes in their cognitive functioning, then we bring in a partner, or cognitive "coach."

Now, the real challenge of this approach, is not the service itself, but in the way and spirit that it is rendered. That is, with the other paradigms reviewed, these kind of supports are seen as maintenance, and the whole spectrum of devaluation follows.

Interdependence promotes that supplemental supports be rightfully, and readily available to the person with the support needs. Further these services should be rendered in an up-beat, and non-aversive way.

I have a friend who directed a "think tank" in Pennsylvania, who has a nice way of talking about the spirit of supplemental supports. When he talks about attendant services, he likens the approach the attendant should take to the person they support as that of a butler to their employer. That is, a butler is a dignified support person who shadows his client. They are anticipatory, and deferring, as their employer calls the shot. They rarely call attention to themselves.

For people who may need some cognitive supports, we might think about the partnership concept as a supplemental support. My colleague, Sharon Gretz, helped me to understand how we might rescript the role that traditional case managers play, into that of a partnership. She contends that the typical supports a case manager might render can be accomplished in a partnership. In her work, Sharon has connected with people who might have been candidates for "case management." With an adjustment in style, timing and a starting point of equality, she and other partners have realized a whole forward step of growth. In the transition, Sharon has learned amazing things about communities and neighborhoods. The partners have developed new and enhanced relationships with people at risk. Everyone is a winner.

When you think about it, the idea of partners makes great interdependence sense. The notion of a case manager implies that people need to be "managed;" that they cannot manage themselves. This implication perpetuates devaluation. Partners, on the other hand, recognize that people might need a hand, but are considered equally in the transaction. All of us have partners in our lives. It's an everyday occurrence. The use of partners for cognitive reinforcement is a viable supplemental support.

Achieving supplemental supports offers a whole new challenge to the rehabilitation agenda. Since supplemental services can be associated with the maintenance paradigm, they are usually difficult to fund. That is, funding sources have considered supplemental supports as custodial and not seen as tied to rehabilitation or growth. Where we have had funding success, such as in Pennsylvania for attendant services, the battle was won not on the merit of rights or viability of service. Rather, we won attendant services in Pennsylvania based on cost savings and deinstitutionalization. Legislators supported it because they thought it would save money.

Another barrier to achieving supplemental supports is related to the economic paradigm. In a simple sense, it is just not worth giving any service to people who are perceived to be less valuable, unless it saves money, or creates a tax base, as with vocational rehabilitation.

These two hurdles, among others, remain in the way of achieving supplemental supports, yet the viability of the service

is real. People should not have to do or be what they are incapable of doing or being, no matter how noble. Rather, we need
to convince the community and system, that the presence of
people who have some difference about them is valuable to the
fabric of community and sometimes supplemental supports are
necessary to make that presence a reality. Unlike homogeneity,
the diversity of people in our midst promotes an openness and
Interdependence that is healthy to us all.

ACTION 3

Relationship Building

☞

*True friendship
comes when silence
between two people is
comfortable.*

D.T. Gentry

If there is a single dimension that must be repeated and
underscored with interdependence, it is that of relationships.
Our daily contacts with others are what makes our lives rich.
Just think of your typical day; the people you touch, the people
that touch you. It boggles the mind. Yet, without them, how
lonely life would be.

As mentioned in Chapter 1, most people with disabilities are
distantiated from typical, freely-given relationships. I know too
many people who only relate with human service professionals
who are paid to be with them.

I have to believe that this is not caused by an absence of
potential recipients of a relationship or because some people do
not possess the skills for relationships, but because we have not
adequately connected or represented people in the community.

Quite simply, members of the community are under the
impression that people with disabilities are just fine in their own
world. Further, as this concept develops, human service workers may be perpetuating the myth. To this point, I have had
professionals boldly tell me, "Come on Al, do you believe that
there are typical people who would choose to be a friend to a
person with a severe disability!"

It is outrageous that people with this notion are in human
services. Can you imagine the audacity and baggage of this
statement? We need to reflect and ask, what creates the real
problem in this relationship issue? If we question the viability of
people with disabilities in obtaining and retaining freely-given
relationships with people who do not have a disability, then I
say - WE ARE PART OF THE PROBLEM! If we perceive that the
key to the relationship problem is found in needing to teach
people with disabilities relationship skills, then I need to ask us
to reassess. Many people who have disabilities may never learn
the "appropriate skills."

We need to pause here, and reflect further on this issue of
relationships with non-disabled people. Recognize, that most

people with disabilities are probably caught up in a homogeneous world, surrounded by other people with disabilities. Since most friendships need the fuel of proximity, and people with disabilities are thrust upon each other, relationships between people with disabilities abound. They seem normal, and often support people promote them and think they are "cute."

Not only can this be demeaning, but it can be atypical in the promotion of relationships. Now it is true that most of us develop relationships from a basic sense of homogeneity. We probably grew up in a town where most of our neighbors and classmates were socioeconomically and culturally similar. As we aged, our relationship experiences probably diversified. To this extent, we started to meet and connect with people with differences.

As these experiences matured, this diversity brings an interesting enrichment to our lives. That is, as we met and related to different people, in an unconscious way we started to place ourselves in the scheme of life. This type of comparison allows us to stretch our awareness of self and life.

Think now about people who have no actual chance to relate to different people, and are constantly in the company of those with disabilities. What a narrow and limited perspective. Yet, in many regards, this is exactly the world we have created for people with disabilities.

Interdependence promotes diversity in relationship opportunities. To this extent, people with disabilities and those without disabilities are encouraged to connect. Indeed, the more exposure people with disabilities have to people without disabilities, the quicker a realization of interdependence.

Now, this notion of homogeneity and heterogeneity are interesting to consider in interdependence. We know that homogeneity does good things for people. For most of us, our security base starts from a sense of being around people who are similar. Certainly, the security levied in our family situations underscores this point.

I know that for me, the security of family is deeply etched. Indeed, living in a small town outside of Pittsburgh surrounded by fifteen families of relatives. It is a true extended family. I know for certain that when the chips are down, I have a whole clan outside my door who know, and care about me.

Yet, if I spent all my time with just my family, I feel my growth would be stagnated as a person. As it stands now, I am extremely fortunate to have the opportunity to travel and experience a wide range of people and situations. This heterogeneous exposure is not only exciting, but vital to my growth. In fact, I believe this mixture of similarity and diversity are opposite members of the same family of growth. Having just one, at the expense of the other, can create a real imbalance.

When I think of the challenge of interdependence, and the issue of homogeneity and heterogeneity, I am drawn by an interesting blend of the concepts. That is, in looking to link people, the homogeneous piece I see is the commonality of interests. This gets back to the issue of "tickets." Each of us has a myriad of interests that are "tickets" to relationships. They might be music, or sports, or poetry. They are common things we share with others, even though we may be very different people in other ways.

I have a friend named Bill. Years ago, he had a head injury and was institutionalized. When we met Bill, most everyone had given up on him. He had little family involvement, and was considered a "behavior problem." He had become very isolated from people.

Our organization in Pittsburgh helped him move into an apartment in the community. Although Bill didn't have that much in common with most people, one ticket he did have was in his love of scripture. Bill spent hours reading the Bible.

Now clearly, there are many people who are interested in scripture. Although these people were different from Bill in background and experience, their homogeneity was found in the Bible. Once the link was made, Bill was on his way to a variety of relationships that continue today.

It is important to underscore here, the spread effect described in Chapter 1. Just as a positive image of a flag positioned near a political candidate can spread the concept of patriotism, so too can value and importance be spread in relationships.

To this point, the more people who might be devalued have opportunity to relate with valued people in communities, the quicker their value will be enhanced. Indeed, think about someone you admire. Now add to that mental picture that person relating with someone who is not as valuable. All of a sudden, the second person's stock will go up. This is particularly true for people with severe disabilities who link with valued people in their community.

A simple adage of this concept takes me back to my mother's advice. Hang around with losers, and you'll tend to become a loser. On the other hand, hang around with winners, you have a greater chance of becoming a winner. Trite, I know, but accurate.

It's not that you always become like those around you, but clearly, you can be influenced. Further, what people think of you is often gauged by who they see you with. Taking this notion to an interdependence perspective, there are two important themes.

One is that homogeneity breeds homogeneity, and that diversity opportunities are extremely limited in homogeneous situations. Yet, diversity is vital to our self-image and enrichment.

Two is that relationships create a spread effect. If we relate with people who are valued, we will tend to be valued. Conversely, if we relate with people who are devalued, we will become, or remain devalued.

To this extent, interdependence recommends actions to facilitate as many opportunities as possible for distantiated people to connect with everyday citizens. This focus alone, however, begins to radically shift the role and actions of support people. Rather than attempt to change people, or speak for them, Interdependence suggests that we function more as bridge-builders.

Bridge-building is a concept that has been explored by a number of forward-thinking social planners associated with the developmental disabilities field. Their ideas are helpful and instructive to interdependence.

Bridge-Building

He who would be a leader, let him first become a Bridge.

Motto from Wales College

Bridge-building, as a term, refers to the connection of distantiated people back to their communities. It is a notion that is much akin to the oriental concept of Shibumi, the blending of similarity and complexity. A bridge is a complex, engineered design to meet a simple need, getting from point A to point B.

In one aspect of bridge-building (Mount, Beeman, & Ducharme, 1988) five key elements are outlined as critical. These are:

❖ *Finding people's interests, preferences, and gifts*

This is an action of uncovering the person's capacities and interests. All people, no matter the severity of situation, have things to add, offer, or contribute.

❖ *Uncovering networks and asking people*

Here, the bridge-builder must map the community and find generic resources that relate to the person's capacities and gifts. Then he must ask people to get involved. Beth Mount stresses the generic aspect, because then there is greater chance for diversity.

❖ *Trusting and letting go*

According to the experts, many connections are missed because the support person cannot let go of fears and concerns. The bridge-builder must be willing to trust and let go. A key to this point is a conscious awareness of how we feel about the person we support and the people we connect them with.

❖ *Using imagination*

Bridge-building is about creativity. There are no prescriptions or cookbooks to follow. This fact pushes us to look beyond our current paradigm and to reach further.

❖ *Accepting uncertainty*

Finally, bridge-building is about connecting and letting go. In this process, the right to risk is actualized. There are no guarantees that the connection will work.

In an exciting way, the concept of bridge-building is a way to interdependence. For the practitioner, it offers a viable way to move from our current, expert-driven thrust, to the role of partner. Perhaps its greatest contribution, however, is that it offers the professional a tangible role to play in achieving Interdependence.

Another important dimension in relationship-building revolves around the levels and stages of relationships. The term, *relationship* can mean many different things. If we are to promote relationship-building in our work, we need to have a clearer understanding of the term.

Relationship is defined by *The Random House Dictionary* as:

1. A connection, association or involvement.
2. A connection between persons by blood or marriage.
3. An emotional or other connection between people: the relationship between teachers and students.
4. A sexual involvement; affair.

For the purposes of interdependence, I define a relationship as the coming together of two people toward a common agenda. This agenda could be as basic as an interest in a hobby, to as complex as forging a life together. To this extent, I see the layering of relationships as follows:

❖ *Basic Acquaintance* – This is the most simple form of relationship. It is merely an acquaintance, or casual connection that is more than a stranger. This might be a person who is in a class you take, and see each week. You nod, or say hello, perhaps some small talk, but no more.

❖ *Focused Acquaintance* – In this relationship, the person is more than a casual connection. At this level, the person is one you feel more attached to. This is the person in your class that you trade quips with, or perhaps occasionally ride home. You know each other's name, some minor details, but no real substance.

❖ *Friend* – At his level, the person now has garnered some level of trust and respect. You feel comfortable connecting with this person outside of the context of how you met. There are clearly some dimensions of this person that are attractive to you.

❖ *Special (Favored) Friend* – As the friendship evolves, this level represents a station of specialness. Time and energy has fused a relationship that is somewhat intense and binding. This is the person you call when the chips are down. Further, this is a person that you feel safe with, confidential information can be transmitted.

❖ *Basic Intimate* – In this category, the relationship has become intimate and highly trusting. Love starts to enter the picture, and the depth of acceptance creates an intensity that is hard to break.

❖ *Focused Intimate* – At this level people are ready to make long standing commitments to each other. Although this can play out in marriage, or contractual bonds, friendships can also forge to this level.

❖ *Covenant* – These relationships are of the deepest nature. They are often bound by lifetime commitments and usually include a vow. Covenant relationships are often associated with the clergy.

Given these levels of relationships, it is important to appreciate the way relationships start, grow, and conclude. Clearly this is a developmental process that requires time and nurturing. They also require proximity, safe ways to grow and input from both parties. Like a strong plant, they require time.

Knowing these things, interdependence suggests that as we focus on relationship building and take into account the dimensions and physical nature of relationships. People may need some support, information, or preparation.

ACTION 4

Systems Advocacy

The final action for interdependence revolves around systems advocacy. Without question, the expert-oriented paradigms reviewed in Chapter 2 have cut a deep line in our system. Laws, regulations, agencies and procedures have been designed around them.

To explore roles, develop supports, promote relationships without equal attention to systems changes is tantamount to a successful day of sailing, only then to miss the harbor upon your return. In fact, more frustrating is that the strides of the previous three dimensions (role enhancement, supplemental supports, and relationship-building) can be totally compromised if we don't spend equal attention on the need for systems change.

Advocacy can carry a number of different definitions. *The Random House Dictionary* defines advocacy as "the act of pleading for, supporting, or recommending; active espousal." To me, advocacy is the action of promoting or advancing a cause. This promotion can be something specific to your situation, or a cause that is important to you. That is, you can work toward something that may have direct benefit to you, or for a cause that directly affects others.

Usually in advocacy, people are more driven by those things that have a direct affect on them. Crime in the neighborhood, or change in a tax law are examples of things that might have direct effect on the advocate's life. Other causes, however, ones that may be indirect to the advocate can stir up as much energy. Examples here might be support to an oppressed group, or actions directed to animals or the environment.

I know some people who argue that all advocacy is really driven by self-interest, even indirect actions. They contend that self-interest is clear when people do something that has direct benefit to them. When they speak out in behalf of an oppressed group, they are demonstrating a clear principle of Interdependence. That is, when any group is oppressed, such as people with disabilities, and we are driven to support causes that have direct benefit to them, we are really moving to shore up our own situation. If any group of people can become (or are) oppressed, then all of us are vulnerable to oppression.

Regardless of motive, or beneficiary, there are clearly some vital elements to advocacy that I believe are essential to making a difference. These are:

Passion	Presence
Position	Perseverance

In my experience, these four elements are critical to advocacy success. They are especially important when the advocacy intent is broad and challenging, as social causes are. It is prudent to review these issues.

Passion

Passion is an emotional term. It is one that conjures up a sense of love, devotion, fire, energy. People who are passionate are said to be intense, and driven by the root of their passion. It might be love, or a job, or a cause.

I believe that passion is the starting point for social advocacy, that without an intense drive, we probably won't get out of the starting block. Much as in love, passion for a cause means a fire has started to burn. The person becomes convinced that the cause is needed in their life, or in their community/society.

Now this lighting of the fire is an interesting notion. Most strong causes, especially those that are social in nature, require someone, or something to light the fire. It might be an incident, or a person that gets the ball rolling. Something causes the fire.

For people susceptible to oppression, the fire can be lit the first time injustice occurs. For others at the direct point of oppression, it might take more time, or multiple experiences. Think of my friends, Tom and Harry, and the story with which I opened this book with. Tom was (and is) a fighter. His fire was lit a long time ago. Harry is more tolerant. In a cerebral way he has come to grips with oppression as his plight in life. Different people come from different spots.

For those not directly subjected to oppression, there may need to be some outside person to ignite a passion. Often it takes a charismatic person to bring these people around. If you examine situations or movements where people have been engaged such as civil rights, the women's movement, the anti apartheid struggle in South Africa, there have been the Kings, Steinems, and Mandelas. All of these leaders have been said to have charisma, or that special ability to influence people.

When we think of charisma, however, there can be a double-edged sword. Just as the charismatic leader can entice people to their movement, they can also become dominant to a point where others in the movement get dwarfed.

In *The Long Haul*, Myles Horton (1990) said of charisma, "The only problem I have with movements has to do with my reservations about charismatic leaders. There's something about having one that can keep democracy from working effectively. But we don't have movements without them. That's why I had no intellectual problem supporting Martin Luther King as a charismatic leader." So passion is the first vital element of advocacy. People need to become engaged and enraged to pick up the cause. Yet, it is important that we understand that passion need not be loud, effective cheerleading. Some of the most passionate advocates I know are quiet, soft-spoken people.

Position

Although passion gets us started on the road to advocacy, it is position that sets the course. Position is the stand we take on the injustice that arouses our passion. That is, if difficulty in entering a building lights our fire, then our position might be architectural accessibility for people with disabilities. If the start point is educational segregation, our position would be mainstreamed schools. If the start point is unemployment, our position might be supported employment programs.

Position is not necessarily the opposite of the root of the passion, although it could be. It is, however, essential to specify the details of the position. That is, loosely defined positions can be nebulous and difficult to focus. The more detailed and specific, the easier to articulate and coordinate with your people.

Another element of position, is that it be realistic and achievable. To let people set out on a course, only to become frustrated, is the easiest way to burn people out. Our positions must be reachable.

This is not to say that we set aside large and noble goals. Rather, I suggest that we develop viable stepping stones to these larger goals. Indeed, we might have multiple positions that lead to an overall goal.

It also helps if our position is generic enough to attract the broadest number of people. This is essential if we are looking to change formal systems. Quite simply, the more people who can be enlisted to support your position, the quicker your group will achieve the position.

Getting consensus on position is not an easy task. People always have opinions, and their opinions are colored by their own situation. Of course, they are going to push for something that is related to their own needs.

So, doing systems work within the interdependent paradigm means that we must become comfortable with consensus building. Much as in politics, we need to incorporate these consensus dimensions to position building. Some get exactly what they wanted, others a little less, but everyone moves forward on common ground. In your looking to address injustice, think about the linking points of your issue to the connection with others.

Obviously, interdependence holds that heterogeneity is a

positive element for communities. Thus, the more people are free to become a part of community, the better the community will be. This point in some ways is paradoxical. That is, as much as heterogeneity may be desirable, the differences of people may make consensus that much more difficult to achieve.

Yet consensus can be reached around broader points of similarity. In spite of physical or cognitive differences of people, the similarity around wanting to participate in community, or in being a part of society is something everyone can relate to. These points of wanting to participate, or be a part of society allows for a basic feature of consensus.

Recently, a friend told me about a linking of two agendas toward a common goal. It was about the Eco-Feminist movement. Here, people looking to advance women's issues had linked up with the ecology movement, forging an interesting amalgamation. The feminists got a diverse area to rally, to show that they can do things beyond the type cast. The ecologists got a strong boost to their numbers allowing them to take on new projects. Both groups were winners. This is a smart lesson in consensus building.

Another example of building consensus was found in a conference held a few years ago between the aging and disability movements. Titled "Unifying the Agenda," people from the independent living movement and the Grey Panthers came together to find common ground. This conference produced an exciting document that is available through the World Institute on Disability (1986).

So to make change, we must advocate a position. This position should be realistic, viable, and hopefully connectable to a larger body of people.

Presence

An organizer for a free society must be a creative person.

S. Alinsky

Once we have articulated a solid and defensible position for our cause, the real work starts. That is, we need to forge strategies to advance our position and be present to see them happen. This means being there.

Certainly, there are many types of strategies and tactics to get a systems point across. Traditional activities have included letters, position papers, rallies, legislative meetings, phone calls, introduction of bills, letters to the editor, public service announcements, press releases, opposite editorials, talk shows, and on and on.

All of these methodologies have been found to be effective in one way or another. Of course, the position will often dictate the strategy, and movements need to be sensitive to things that have worked, and have not worked.

A presence can also be had in some untraditional ways. Most often this means a gimmick, or something that influences beyond logic. An interesting current example of an untraditional approach is the AIDS Quilt. This massive effort is a weaving together of 4x4 sections of cloth lovingly and sensitively adorned with inscriptions and messages by family and friends to those taken by AIDS. In a powerful and visible way, this quilt has drawn more attention than most traditional approaches.

Other nontraditional ways include films, walks, concerts, and plays. One such example was the "Hands Across America" effort held a few years ago to draw attention to the issues of homelessness. This event endeavored to field a human chain, hand by hand, across America.

A powerful, nontraditional, and permanent effort toward attention to a problem of distantiation is found with the Vietnam Veterans Memorial in Washington, D.C. This architectural wonder has touched more people than was ever intended.

And so, when we consider a presence to our position, the sky is the limit. We must, however, be cautious about "events" or activities that may tend to devalue, or negatively image our cause.

To this point, I am drawn by a section of the quarterly magazine, *The Disability Rag*. For those of you who do not know, the *Rag* has emerged as the consciousness of the disability movement. Their motto is, "read the *Rag* and think." Each edition has a feature, "Things we wish we wouldn't see." Invariably, this section exposes or highlights campaigns, fund raising, public awareness, and other methods used by agencies and organizations to bring public attention to disability issues. Usually, these ads are pity-oriented or schmaltzy beyond belief.

When we think of presence then, let's remember that the end does not justify the means. Indeed, during the period of the "means," many an attitude gets forged. We need to be present, but we must be conscious and aware of our actions.

Perseverance

The final message of systems advocacy is found in perseverance. Any social movement worth its salt, does not happen overnight. Awareness and attitude shift happens slowly and tediously. It's real easy to get impatient. To this extent, Interdependence demands, much as Myles Horton described in his book, that we are in for a long haul. We need to find ways and means to persevere.

As we look at perseverance and other movements, there are some instructive actions. One is that we remember to always look to add new people to our cause. Often, movements can

ॐ

There must be a beginning to any great matter, but the continuing into the end until it be thoroughly finished yields the true glory.

Sir Francis Drake

become elitist. People get so wrapped up in the cause, that they forget to bring others along.

This notion is interesting because it ties in ego and celebrity. That is, those at the core of a movement tend to become the spokespeople. As the movement takes on steam, the spokespeople move to the front, and then into the limelight. This spot not only feels good, but can become seductive. You know the old saying about power corrupting. Well, it can and does happen in movements. The way we can guard from this happening is to be sure we talk about it, share the limelight, and constantly bring in new people.

Another important consideration is celebration. So often, our causes are serious and intense. We can get so caught up in this mindset, that we forget to celebrate. We need to insure that we take opportunity to recognize this point.

One great way to celebrate is through food and song. There is something magical when people eat or sing together. It has an uplifting, spiritual thrust. When you break bread, or sing, you bond, and any movements need bonding.

Over the years, as I have had the opportunity to travel and talk with people about interdependence, I have had a real chance to observe how groups address this issue. In this awareness, I am always struck by the spirit and soul I find in Canada. For a number of reasons, I find people in Canada more gentle and spiritual than we in America. I think the thing that drives this home, however, is found in the issues of song and food and celebration.

During one of my early visits to Canada, I remember sitting around in the hospitality room, eating and singing, well after the conference sessions were concluded. One person had an accordion (which happens to be one of my favorite instruments; it must have something to do with my Italian genes), another, a tambourine, and we sang. All were welcome.

Somehow, this scene of people with an accordion and tambourine would not happen in the typical American gatherings and conferences I attend. It seems that people are too preoccupied with other agendas. These agendas permeate and often people are found marketing or impressing each other. It seems we all do it. That is why I go to Canada every chance I get. It's just a different tone.

This is not to say that spirit and soul cannot be found in America. Indeed, I recently attended a retreat held at the Highlander Center in Tennessee. After all the reading I had done and the "movement" history that is etched at Highlander, I was delighted to spend time there. What I found was an amazing sense of spirit.

To sit in a rustic circular room, on rocking chairs with the Smoky Mountains as a backdrop — believing the Highlander philosophy that says that people know the solution to their problems, all they need is the space — is a wonderful experience. We sat, thought, talked, ate, sang and stayed together for three days. Not only did we make progress in our issue for the retreat, but we forged a powerful spirit that will help us carry it through.

A final aspect to perseverance is pace. Often our intensity and commitment to change, causes us to push as many buttons as we can, as quickly as we can. This is a fast track to burnout. We would all do better to think through a longer plan. This not only prolongs our presence, but also doesn't abuse our people.

Now, as we talk about this, it is important in our pacing not to miss opportunities, or to bore our people. Pace is an art. You can do it too fast, or too slow. Think about balance. Take readings from your people. Watch for the signposts of burnout.

So, there we have it. Achieving interdependence is not an easy task, but there are some directions we can take. We need to remember in the four aforementioned activities, role competency enhancement, supplemental supports, relationship building, and systems advocacy, must all blend together. One area is no more important than another.

Further, all of this must emanate from the person with a disability at the core. They must have the freedom to define their problems, and be in the lead with the solutions. This means that the present roles that have emerged from our expert driven paradigms must shift. The power must be transitioned from the expert to the consumer.

When I discuss interdependence with audiences that perceive themselves as experts, this concept of a power shift is hard to ingest. First, the experts voice concern that the consumers will not make good decisions without them. Then they softly voice concern about their jobs.

To this first notion, there is no question that some people with disabilities who take control over their lives may not have the best of decision-making skills. Some will, some will not. Interdependence does not suggest that people be cast into the sea without oars. Rather, we all need to figure out how viable supplemental supports can be introduced that will meet this need. Much as attendant services have liberated people with physical disabilities from institutions, so too can cognitive supports do the same for people with challenges in decision making.

I think, however, that the cognitive supports are best when naturally developed in relationships. That is, rather than people being denied control, or regulated by experts, I believe that when people are connected to other people in community in real ways, supports will follow. Now certainly, these relationships have to be cultured and nurtured, but they are possible.

As for the job security issue, I believe that professionals will still have an important role in the shift to interdependence. Of course, the role will change, but not end; at least in the near future. Rather than function as experts who assess and treat, I see professionals as the persons who connect and support.

However, in this new role, it becomes imperative that professionals understand and know community. We cannot effectively connect people, or find alternatives, unless we have a viable working knowledge of community. So, although there are things to say about the professional's role in a paradigm shift to Interdependence (and I plan to write more on this in the future), a more pressing reality for this book is to introduce community.

PERSONAL AND ORGANIZATIONAL CHALLENGES

Over the years, as I have understood and shared ideas related to interdependence, the most perplexing question, one that stands well over the others previously mentioned, is where do we start? Understanding, accepting and agreeing with Interdependence is all well and good, but this concept will never happen unless first steps are taken.

As I have thought about first steps, like most other aspects of interdependence, there are two streams of change — personal and organizational that must be considered. Although these two dimensions can be considered separately, they really must happen together. You cannot have organizational change, unless you have a majority of people in the organization who accept, respect and allow change. Similarly, you cannot have personal change unless the organization allows you to explore and flirt with new ideas. To a certain extent, this means organizational openness. It also means personal openness.

Let's examine both fronts.

❖ *Personal Change* – I am always intrigued by people who are inspired to explore and reflect on new ideas. What causes these entrepreneurs to be open and flexible to new ideas?

Obviously this is a major area of psychological thought and reflection. In most cases we attribute change to people who have the following attributes or factors associated with their situation:

secure	flexible
restless	creative
happy	open
unhappy	experimental

Each of these dimensions alone are subjects of countless books, essays and reflections. Indeed, psychological tests have been developed to help gauge, or predict what people are prone to these various characteristics.

It is not the intent of this book to necessarily turn people into entrepreneurs.

In fact, if you have gotten this far in this book, I think you probably have the major elements of change in your character. One of the readers of this manuscript joked that *Interdependence* should be a litmus test for openness and tolerance as very deep rooted paradigms are challenged.

Suffice it to say, that if something in the pit of your gut tells you that things can be better in human services; that persons who have disabilities can be in the community; that you do not have to be sick to get better; then you have the juice to start forward in a quest for continued personal and organizational change.

Here are some ideas to promote and nurture your openness to change. I offer them as tips, thoughts and options that have worked for me and others that I admire and respect.

❖   *Read* – Simple as it might seem, I'm amazed at how easy it is for people to drift from reading. Take time, find it, make it, steal it, however, but take time to read. Never dismiss anything that comes across your desk. Read as much as you can about human services, or items that relate in any way to human services. Along with the main text, for me, some of the most exciting aspects of a book or article is the bibliography, or reference list. I see these entries as a map to further understanding the concept or topic of the article. Know, that most items you read will reference ways and means to more basics from its paradigmatic roots. The reference list will guide you to these roots.

     The bibliography from this book, for example, is full of wonderful books and articles that have been essential to my synthesis. Although each is focused to its particular topic in one way or another I see these writings as the grains of interdependence. They are all seeds to my understanding of change. Know too, that some of my references are off the beaten track, but when you're searching for answers, clues are often found in out of the way places.

❖   *Reflect* – No amount of reading produces a really electric change unless you reflect on it. This reflection can happen immediately after reading, or can occur many days later. By reflection, I mean the conscious review and realization of what was read.

     Often if I am struck by something, I will jot it on a note card. Additionally, I always underline and make notations in my books. Not only does this allow me to easily go back to passage that need further reflection, but these markings serve to remind and push people who borrow my books to return them. They feel too guilty to keep something that has been personally marked.

Study passages that are provocative, for or against your cause. Read them out loud, listen and think about their meaning as it relates to your paradigm.

It should be noted here, that people typically do not often read, or reflect on writings that refute or challenge their paradigms. That is, liberals tend to read liberal writings, and conservatives, theirs; yet the best routes to personal change are not when an agenda is confirmed — but when a thesis is challenged. This provocation pushes you to examine and defend your position. I've had many personal experiences when my initial beliefs could not hold up under a new challenge. This caused me to either shore up my thinking or to change.

❖ *Reflect with others* – It is one thing to dissect an idea by yourself, and quite another to spar with a friend. In this suggestion, I am not recommending that you become a polished debater. Rather, that you explore interesting or provocative pieces or passages with people you respect or enjoy.

One thing we have done in Pittsburgh is to develop a "book club." This group of six to eight people meets regularly to read and then discuss books or chapters. We usually gather over dinner and nourish both our minds and bodies. Great discussions abound.

Although most reflections typically occur with those we like and share a paradigm with, efforts should be made to explore ideas with those who may come from a different angle. These discussions are "harder," but are ones that tend to expand thinking.

Indeed, personal change is a private matter. People have to be ready to change. In other situations, outside variables can push people to change. Regardless the process of change can be painful, frightening and nerve racking. For many the sheer idea of doing something different can create terror.

On the other hand, change can also be exciting exhilarating and liberating. It can open new doors that enhance and sweeten life.

In spite of this virtual paradox of emotions and feelings associated with change, this review of ways to promote personal change has been a cursory one. There have been excellent books, articles and monographs that have explored personal change in detail.

For my thesis on interdependence however, once persons are ready to make a move, a key struggle comes with organizational change. How can we get groups of people, many who have been set in their paradigm, to think about new ways and to consider change. Remember, most agents of organizations have been deeply committed to their paradigm. They have paid long and hard "dues" to get in. Further, most organizations have a deeply embedded history that relates to the *status quo* and the way things always have been done in the "industry." May organizations are reluctant to change what they perceive to be a winning game.

This gets us back to the risk associated with change. If some individuals within an organization feel change is necessary, this perception may not be accepted or embraced by colleagues. If the new agenda is pushed too fast and too assertively, others, even those at the cusp of change might pull back. This interface between personal change and organizational change is fragile at best.

Regardless of this fragility, there are some organizational actions that can help with the process of change. Once enough people are ready to hear and act, there are some steps to take in a process to guide organizational change. Let me share a process that has worked for me.

ORGANIZATIONAL CHANGE

As interdependence is such a holistic concept, those of us so inclined realize that change can and should happen on a number of fronts. Our families, neighborhoods, communities, churches, and places of employment are all settings and/or organizations that can be influenced. Some of the components of organizational change can occur in any or all of these settings.

When I discuss the tenets of interdependence, however, it is the organization or system that creates human services that cause the greatest discussion. That is, many people interested in interdependence say to me, "This is a great concept but how do I apply it to my organization? How do I make it happen in my agency?"

Often these questions are awkward, because they suggest the experts should decide; that someone else will know all the answers. Yet, I, or people like me am not necessarily expert on your organization. In fact, I struggle with the ways and means to interdependence with my own agency, UCP of Pittsburgh.

I can however, share some ideas or steps to change that have been viable to our struggle in Pittsburgh. For the past few years, we have been trying to come to grips with interdependence and to make it work for us. This effort has been invigorating yet, at

times, slow and tedious. It is vital to keep in mind that continued forward progress on the process is as important as the end
goal.

As I reflect on our attempts at organizational change, there
have been strategic steps that have been helpful to us. Here are
those steps.

1. Articulate the mission

Most organizations have a mission statement. This is a
succinct and concise overview of what the organization hopes to
accomplish. I believe that it is not enough to attempt to teach,
or rehabilitate people. A solid mission statement must express
the context to a large extent, the ultimate goal.

Here is the mission statement we articulated at UCP:

> *The mission of UCP (United Cerebral Palsy of the Pittsburgh
> District) is to support people with disabilities as they explore
> options, participate in the community and strive toward equality.
> In short, working toward a community where each belongs.*

Now, the importance of the mission statement must be
underscored. This statement is the core of the organization; it is
why it is in business. Everything around the organization
should support the accomplishment of this statement.

When UCP realized the need to shift from an expert model to
interdependence we called a retreat to review and adjust our
mission statement. This two-day gathering included people who
had used, or were currently using our services, a range of staff,
and board members. We brought in an outside facilitator and
hammered out our statement.

The process was not easy; there was debate and key differences that had to be resolved. Yet, at the end of the two days we
had a vital document, one to which we could all commit.

What about your organization? Do you have a clear and
concise mission statement? Does it reflect what you feel is
needed? Does it indeed, reflect what you actually do?

If you find confusion or discourse in answering these questions upon review of your document, your organization has
some basic work to do. This doesn't mean your organization is
not viable, or helpful. Rather it may call attention to the drifting
reality of the day, or the extent to which things have passed you
by.

2. List out guiding principles

The most important factor, to organizational change, I
believe, is for your organization to identify guiding principles to
accomplish your mission. The guiding principles are just that,

key statements that should guide and influence all organizational decisions. They are short, succinct parameters that serve to keep the organization anchored to its paradigm.

With interdependence, these principles are the cornerstone to keep the organization on track. They also offer a real point of comparison to evaluate and reflect on past action. In a sense, they can keep the organization ethically consistent.

In Pittsburgh, we etched out our principles at the same retreat where we clarified our mission. The principles we subscribe to are as follows:

1. We support the uniqueness, wholeness and dignity of each person. We shall strive to respond to the individual needs and preferences of each person we support and serve.

2. We enthusiastically advocate for the rights of people with disabilities so they may fully participate in and contribute to community life. This includes enjoying a secure home, family, friends, education, services and work they find meaningful.

3. We view all human life as having equal and unconditional value. Each life should be nurtured, respected, celebrated and fulfilled.

4. We support the life-long process of personal growth and development of all people.

5. We will take every opportunity to educate others and to advocate for the basic civil rights of people with disabilities:

   — *The right to prevention, early diagnosis and proper care.*
   — *The right to a barrier-free environment and accessible transportation.*
   — *The right to an appropriate public education.*
   — *The right to necessary assistance, given in a way that promotes independence.*
   — *The right to a choice of lifestyles and residential alternatives.*
   — *The right to an income for a lifestyle comparable to the able-bodied.*
   — *The right to training and employment as qualified.*
   — *The right to petition social institutions for just and humane treatment.*
   — *The right to self-esteem.*

UCP BILL OF RIGHTS

6. We emphasize cooperation in getting things done through and with the people we serve.

7. We vigilantly adhere to these values.

I must admit that keeping to these principles is a task. Often we slip back to "old ways" and forget the inclusive and cooperation we stated are vital. Usually, however, someone on our leadership team will call us back and we will ground ourselves. Sometimes, at our meetings, we will put the principles up on the flip chart as an active reminder.

As you think about the principles that guide your organization, recognize that this is where the greatest opportunity to promote interdependence lies. Know too, that this is also the point of greatest threat and resistance. Just a discussion of guiding principles will tell you where people are "at," in your organization.

Keep in mind that some people on your leadership team will want to develop guiding principles, others may not. Some may want to promote principles that seemingly work against interdependence.

Thus, prior to this step in the process, you must be sure that most of your colleagues, up and down the organizational scale, are ready for change. To move too soon in this stage could literally push your agency further into its existing paradigm, than out into interdependence.

If you sense your agency is not ready to address guiding principles, your efforts toward change should not stop, but merely adjust. Resistance to this process suggests that people need more "values" input that promote interdependence. Books like this one, and others referenced, should be passed around your team. Try to promote opportunities for people to talk about these concepts. Staff meetings and training opportunities present a good opportunity to reflect. Another thought is to suggest that an outside person, familiar with Interdependence be invited to spend time at your agency. These are all ways to promote a dialogue toward interdependence.

3. List out strategies to achieve the mission

At this point, if you have developed a succinct mission statement, and guiding principles have been detailed, your organization is now ready to review and brainstorm strategies to achieve the mission. In this process, of course, present strategies, programs and actions should be tested. Other ideas, however, should be identified and included. A key in the process is to list every and any way that the mission might be achieved. Don't worry at this point, if the ideas cost too much, or if the staff aren't trained, or if the board isn't ready. These are all points of clarification that will occur later. For now, you don't want to miss a beat.

There are many different ways to brainstorm. Some groups have used "Story boarding", a Disney initiated way to promote maximum creativity. Usually a trained facilitator is needed to do "Story boarding" the right way.

Another process, one that I like to use, is a "nominal process" where everyone present writes down a stream of ideas. Then in serial fashion, each idea is listed by the facilitator. Everyone in the process participates and all ideas get recorded and noted.

Regardless of your approach, the process should yield some interesting information. Not only should you generate a lot of good ideas, but, if the guiding principles discussion produced viable interdependence concepts, some listed existing practices that are anchored in the medical paradigm, should jump out. In some regards this process initiates a paradigmatic clarification. If things are done right, you can come to grips with "good" and "bad" practices.

4. Prioritize Strategies

This fourth step is rug-cutting time. This is where the guiding principles meet the options of strategies to present the "road to interdependence".

Of course this is also where the hardest decisions might lie, especially if most of the existing organizational practices are medically driven. Yet, if the process has been followed, and most people on the leadership team understand interdependence and are seeking change, then this is the time to make it happen.

With our experience in Pittsburgh, at this point in the process, some key decisions were made that have led to total reorganization. It became clear that we were concerned about the negative effects of segregative programs driven from a diagnostic focus. Yet up to this point in the process, UCP had been running a diagnostically specific Independent Living Rehabilitation Program designed to teach people with disabilities life skills. Further, we had set up separate tracks within this program for separate disability groups.

As we realized these factors, our organization embarked on some critical adjustments. This change has been designed to de-emphasize disability and diagnosis issues. To do this, we're in the process of developing a community center for personal development. This center will focus on personal development for all people interested in change. Rather than having just services for people with disabilities, our center plans to host a variety of activities for all types of persons interested in personal growth. I anticipate hosting literacy programs, adult education and community college courses in the not too distant future.

Although we will continue to support community opportunities for people with disabilities, this change is a critical step toward achieving a more interdependent focus to our organization. As we move from being known in the community as a place where "handicapped people" go, to a place that promotes and offers personal development opportunities for all people, vital integration should occur. In a way, this is a reverse integration activity. Since it is difficult for us to take people out individually (due to support needs and limited attendant supports available) this change will bring diverse people to our center.

5. Focus action toward best strategies

The fifth step in the process is an action and planning one. This is where the organization sets time frames for the actions and strategies vital to interdependence. In some regards this step can be tricky, especially if the organization decides to shift from one type of service to another. In these situations, deep roots from the old paradigm can be difficult to erase, even when the organization makes a dedicated decision to change.

Further, at this point the organization has the critical task of making sure that funding sources understand the reasons and viability of the change. In fact, keeping the funding sources abreast of change before its ultimate initiation is important to proactive planning. This is particularly true if the planned change is significant. That is, if your program shifts from doing group homes to more integrated apartments and your funding sources are not aware of your change, they might have difficulty when they learn of your shift.

Along with funding sources, it is also important to have fellow agencies in your service network also know of and appreciate your plans to change programming. It is important in this process, however, not to devalue or threaten other programs in this process. They should not be forced to look "bad" as you make their changes. Rather, they need to come to their own decisions for change.

It is important to note, that when people make fundamental changes, especially if they announce the changes are for the better, that people who knew the person prior to the change might feel threatened. Often, a better than thou attitude can accompany change and this attitude can be a "put down" to others in the process.

As we move to make changes with our program in Pittsburgh I often find myself in the awkward spot of describing and defining our reasons to change. Often in this translation colleagues from other agencies tease me. Recently a friend shared that a key human service official in Pittsburgh described me as a "missionary." The implication was that I had seen the "light" and wanted to convert others.

Now, I don't know if I'm a missionary, but I do feel strongly about interdependence. I feel this is a necessary paradigm for human services and that others need to think about its efficacy. If this is being a "missionary", then I guess I am guilty.

6. Evaluate

As with any formal action in human services, evaluation of how things are working is a critical step that many organizations fail to take. Making major changes is never easy, and can often be perverted or altered. The organization making change must constantly be assessing its progress toward the goal.

In this analysis, an important element of evaluation rests with comparing and contrasting change action off the interdependent paradigm. That is, the guiding principles developed in Step 2 play a vital role in the overall evaluation of progress. If the guiding principles have been well constructed, any paradigmatic change can be easily evaluated.

A finale note of evaluation is found with the capacity to adjust once a deviance is uncovered. In the change effort, either personal or organizational barriers and gaps will occur. More than just identifying their presence, true evaluation promotes quick and deliberate corrective action. Without it, evaluation is only half effective.

And so, to have interdependence requires that we change. This change starts with individuals, but does not really become dramatic until it is embraced by organizations. Both individual and organizational changes are incredibly complex, but there are some actions or steps that can offer a start point to this process. This section has presented some personal actions and ideas.

Know, however, that there can be many other ways to personal and organizational change. It is not so important that the ones here be actualized, as it is for you to move forward toward change. Use whatever means works for you, but do something.

5

Understanding Culture and Community

The most important thing we face in the 21st century is a rediscovery of community.

*Willard Gaylin
(World of Ideas)*

5

Understanding Culture and Community

The key to interdependence is found in understanding community. Yet it is amazing to me how little most of us know about culture and communities. We agree that our goal in human services is to reunite people with disabilities to community, still we don't spend much time on the subject. Consider the curriculum you studied in school or conferences and educational gatherings you attend. Probably the majority of time is spent on specifics of disability, how it occurs, manifestations and typical associated deficits. Usually little, or no attention paid to culture or community.

This deficit perspective, of course, is a manifestation of the medical/expert paradigms that functions more as a predictive science. Although the goal of intervention is to get people back to their communities, the paradigm has taught us that the way to this goal is through fixing or changing the person. We have devoted little, or no attention to the world around the person with a disability. It's no wonder that there are often community acceptance issues when we do venture out there.

I feel that today's communities indeed are uncomfortable with people who have disabilities. I believe, however, that this is not due to the people with disabilities themselves, but with the fact that professionals have rushed in to relieve communities of their responsibilities. The net result is that people with disabilities have been extracted and put out of sight.

To understand this, think of the trends. Most communities today seem to have been encouraged to parcel off people, especially those who are perceived to have difficulties to separate settings. Our communities have developed special centers, homes and/or shelters for those who are at risk. Of course, all this development has been driven primarily by professionals and community leaders who purport to care.

Another trend occurring in conjunction with this compartmentalization, is the importation of those to do the caring. That is, many people who run or provide professional services to these people at risk are not native to the community. They usually come into the community during their "work hours," perform some function, and then go back to their home community at the end of the day.

These human service trends did not start with, nor are they continued with any intended maliciousness. Clearly, I think, most human service workers, and the communities that host them, regardless of area of specialty, believe they are doing what is right. They are convinced, mostly by their paradigm of origin, that they are meeting the needs.

In my analysis, though, these actions have altered some of the very essence of what has made our communities unique, the ability to solve their own problems, and the acceptance of diverse people within their midst. As more and more people, however, become seen as needy and different, the trends are for experts to be pulled in to take care of these "problems." This care taking is tantamount to extracting these "problem people" from community.

I liken this trend to what might happen to a piece of cloth. If you think of cloth as a bonding of unique strands, and then begin to pull a strand here, and a strand there from the cloth, before you know, you have a weak and tattered cloth. I think the same is with a culture. If you remove the elderly here, and the poor there, and next people with disabilities, soon you have a weaker community.

Years gone by wasn't like this. I don't consider myself that old, but I can remember my community in the late 50s. This was before specialty agencies and senior citizen centers. People were together, and there seemingly was a place for all.

I particularly remember a fellow by the name of Merle. I'm sure Merle had some type of cognitive disability, but that did not seem to matter in our community. Merle sold papers at the corner of our main street, ran errands, helped with groceries, and always seemed to be the key man at community events, street fairs and the like.

I don't like to be a pessimist, but I am sure if Merle was alive today, he would be in some sheltered workshop and live in a group home. He would have a program plan and a team of therapists trying to make his life better. But you know, I don't think Merle's life could have been better than it was. He was well-known in our town, and had lots of friends. He was somebody.

So to me, it seems human services has hastened to make life better for distantiated people. Yet, with jargon, therapies, and knowledge, these actions might just be making things worse. In fact, Wolf Wolfensberger recently said, that if all human services would end today, the net effect to the lives of people with disabilities would be zero. No better, but no worse.

For some professionals, this might be a hard pill to swallow, but I think Wolfensberger is on to something here. If my friend Merle was not an integral member of our community, both Merle and our community would have been the losers. The bold face of this fact is that sometimes community-oriented human services can be iatrogenic.

DEFINING CULTURE

For our understanding here, I am defining culture as a network of people bound together by some common cause or interest. This definition might differ from some anthropologists and sociologists as being too narrow or parochial. Yet, it seems to me that culture, as a word, can be used in a number of ways. That is, we can speak of an American culture or a European culture and this definition will have a sweeping notion amidst much diversity. Still, my definition would apply to America as much as it would to a church culture, these are networks of people bound by a common cause or interest. For the church example, the common interest is, of course, spirituality. For the example of American culture, it is the common interest that a nation of people have.

Cultures are distinguished by the common rituals, rules, and boundaries. They have either informal or formal leaders and the membership is held constant by at least one prevailing theme that everyone holds dear. New members often have to prove themselves before they are invited to join the culture.

Given this definition, it is important to know that all of us are members of a number of cultures (some might call them subcultures) in the course of our lives. As I think about it, there are some cultural situations common to us all. Consider these:

Family Culture — Perhaps the basic network of people bound by some common cause is the family. All of us start out life and learn the basics of culture through our families. Along with our nuclear family, we all have the larger, extended family that includes all aspects of our genealogy. Most of us have a fair handle on our ancestry and nurture our understanding through photos, stories, and family reunions. I have an interesting lens in which to think about my extended family culture by looking out my living room window. As you know from my previous stories, I live on a family "hill" with 15 other relatives. We see each other daily and are richly nourished by regular interaction. Recently, a local TV station was doing a special on the family and used "Condeluci Hill" as one of their examples. As the reported interviewed the various members of my family, I was impressed by how many of my relatives mentioned the power of our proximity as one of the key reasons we are so strong as a family.

Spiritual Culture — Most sustaining nations are anchored by strong spiritual cultures within their midst. A spiritual culture is a network of people bound together by a common theology. These are usually organized as congregations, parishes, or temples. In some cases, these groups are even more focused through an ethnic tie-in as well. My own spiritual culture, Mother of Sorrows Roman Catholic Church is not only a grouping of Catholics, but the parish is further delineated by its strong Italian heritage as well. At our parish, we celebrate Italian customs as much as we do Catholic ones.

Work Culture — Another network of people bound by some common cause is work group. Most of us have spent some time in our lives as members of a company or organization. In these roles, despite differences we might have in ethnicity, age, religion, or any other variable, we are all similar as employees. Indeed, many companies work hard to create a distinct "work culture" where people can enhance morale by being members of the team. This gets embellished by company logos, nicknames, advertisements, and the like, all designed to promote a loyalty to the culture. Some settings where a union is present can present a real question to the employee. In these cases, who are you loyal to? Your company or the union? In the 1994 professional baseball strike, the loyalty factor was even more compromised. In this situation, you had the ball players who were all members of their team, also pulled by the union, and then ultimately criticized by the fans. Sometimes cultures can have very complex features.

Age Culture — Another delineation that can bond people into a culture is age. In fact, with our educational system set up with age-specific groups, we are all habituated with our age peers. In the news, we hear about the "baby boomer" culture that has influenced all aspects of society. I was amused by all the hoopla given on the Woodstock 94 efforts to capture the peace and love culture of the original Woodstock concert held in 1969. All the chronicles of our society are intrigued by the elements of the age culture. We have stories on "generation X," or the "post-baby boomers" all designed to show how people can be bound in common experience with a network of others.

Neighborhood Culture — People who live in certain areas are also influenced by the common interests and concerns driven by proximity. Most of us are concerned about the physical state of our neighborhood, how it looks, and how it holds its value. Indeed, today, crime and safety in our neighborhoods reigns as the most important issue on the minds of Americans. Some neighborhoods have developed safety patrols, escorts, and other methods to make sure their fellow neighbors are not victimized. These neighborhood groups offer a classic example of a network of people bound by a common territory.

Ethnic Culture — All of us have an ethnic starting point for our families. This bond is so powerful that regardless of any other factor, if you hold ethnic origins with another person, often that commonality can become a strong point of identification. I know in my own situation, as an Italian, many people will approach me and introduce themselves as Italians. In fact, the Italian work "piasan" means brother and is often used as a precourse to an introduction. Many African-Americans refer to each other as "brothers or sisters." Indeed, ethnicity is a strong commonality that bonds a network of people together.

Sex or Sexual Orientation Culture — With the advent of the women's movement in the 60s, we began to see the bonding of people based on their sex. I can remember hearing speeches at NOW meetings where each speaker implored their "sisters" to band together to fight sexual oppression. Just being a woman was the criteria for common bond. Not much later, men's collectives were formed to help men break out of male stereotype roles and discover other parts of their humanity. More recently, men's groups have attempted to connect with their more primal being by spending outdoor time with other men beating drums and pushing closer to their core. Beyond this are the homo-sexual and lesbian cultures, as well as the broader implications of being gay for those who have the common bond of sexual orientation. I have gay friends who talk proudly of the "gay culture."

Common Interest Culture — This catch-all category refers to those networks of people who bond together because of some common interest. This could be people interested in photogra-phy, tennis, poetry, dogs, politics, or countless other advocations that people might find in common. The list is virtually endless, and if you live in a large urban area, it is incredible diversity of the groups that gather. All of these gather-ings are cultures in and of themselves. They have common language, rituals, and rules that they hold dear.

For the purposes of achieving interdependence, we not only need to understand the power and prominence of cultures in our life, but more importantly, we also need to know how these cultures embrace something new. Anthropologists call this "cultural diffusion." Quite simply, cultural diffusion is the process by which a culture comes to assimilate an alien, or alien perspective into the bosom of the culture. For those of us interested in seeing people with disabilities returned to their culture and community, we must come to understand how cultures diffuse new information. Although there is much sophisticated research on this topic, I have discovered some basic elements that I feel can help in our efforts of cultural diffusion. These are:

> *Understand Natural Hesitancies:* As previously mentioned, all cultures have natural boundaries, membership, leadership, rules, regulations, and language. These elements create an offsetting from other cultures. It is natural when something new is introduced to the culture there will be suspicion, and possible rejection. The culture needs to test out the new item before it can truly be embraced.
>
> *Valued Gatekeepers:* The most typical way something new is introduced to a new culture is through a valued gatekeeper. These are the cultural leaders, either formal or informal, who are respected or valued within the culture. The gatekeeper is the person who can open the gates to a culture to adopt or sanction something novel. It is important to know that the gatekeeper may not necessarily be a formal elected or titled leader. It is always, however, the most influential person within the peer group. This is the person who sets the trends, initiates the fads, pushes the culture closer to something new. Think about your own cultures. Who are the gatekeepers you can identify that play this role? I know in my own situations where I find myself in leadership roles, I am quick to try to identify the gatekeeper and enlist them to help me in my cause. I know that these people can influence and I want to be sure that they are working with, rather than against my cultural objectives.
>
> *Woman as Gatekeepers:* In thinking about the role of gatekeeper for the purpose of introducing people who have been devalued back into a culture, I am intrigued by the impact of women. As I have done research, as well as more anecdotal observation, it seems that women reach out more to welcome and introduce devalued people to the group. I am not sure why this is, but clearly women are drawn more to the helping professions and are often more critical in the care giving role. It seems too, that women are more prone to pull for the underdog or feel for the person who loses. This natural propensity is powerful when one considers the job of connecting someone who has been an alien back to the culture. Now, it is more important to know that only current

members of a culture can serve as gatekeepers. No matter how interested you are in seeing someone entered and welcomed into a culture, as an outsider, you will not be able to serve as a gatekeeper. Only current members can play this role. This is where women can play a significant role. That is, if you are trying to assist someone into a new culture, and you are not a member of that culture, then you will need a gatekeeper. If you do not know a member personally, your best bet is to find a woman in the group who might play this role.

There is so much more that could be said about cultures, but we must move on. Often, the word *culture* is used synonymously with the word *community*. Indeed, a culture can be a community and in many ways a community can be defined much as I have done in looking at culture, but there are key differences. Let us examine community.

DEFINING COMMUNITY

Rather then etching out my own definition of community, I have gone to some excellent sources to look at this phenomena. Consider these definitions:

❖ Webster (*Complete Unabridged Dictionary*, 1985): "Community is a unified body of individuals. People with common interest living in a particular area. The area itself. An interacting population of various kinds of individuals. A group of people with a common characteristic or interest living together within a larger society.

❖ Warren and Warren (*The Neighborhood Organizer's Handbook*, 1979): "The community of place – the proximate neighborhood setting - is a vital part of growing up, of raising families, of meeting many of the changes and stresses of urban life."

❖ Hillary, George (*Rural Sociology*, Vol 20, 1955, pp. 194-204) "Community is a group integrated through a system of spatially contingent, interdependent biotic, cultural, and social relations and structure which have evolved in the process of mutual adjustment to environmental situations."

◆ McKnight, John (*Beyond Community Services*, 1988): Communities are collective associations. In a sense, they are more and different than friendship... It is groups of people who work together on a face-to-face basis and are engaged in public rather than private life.

❖ Sussmen, Martin (*Community Structure and Analysis*, 1959) "Community is a human population living in a given geographical area which has interdependence and often specialization of function and which shares a common culture."

❖ Nisbit, Robert (*Quest for Community*, 1972): "Community thrives on self-help, either corporate of individual, and everything that removes a group from the performance of an involvement in its own government can hardly help but weaken the sense of community. People do not come together in significant and lasting associations merely to be together, they come together to do something that cannot easily be done in individual isolation."

❖ O'Brien, John (*Discovering Community*, 1986): "We can promote a sense of community if we develop the competence to overcome our habits of segregation, professionalization, and bureaucratization on even the smallest scale. Discovering community means testing the everyday assumptions of the service world through action and reflection."

❖ O'Connell, Mary (*The Gift of Hospitality*, 1988): "Community is no different for people with disabilities than for any of the rest of us. It is the free space where people think for themselves, dream their dreams, and come together to create and celebrate their community humanity."

As I think about these definitions, I am struck by the notion of consent, creativity, and cooperation, all important ingredients of community. In fact, it was the power of consent and associations that struck Alexis de Tocqueville in his 1883 analysis of America, as written in his haunting book, *Democracy in America*. To de Tocqueville, our propensity to create freely formed associations to deal with issues in our community was what made (and many believe still makes) us great as a country.

Indeed, think about most communities today. If there are needs that crop up, invariably a group or association will form to address the issue. Maybe it's the concern for a littered vacant lot, or a patrol for Halloween night to keep the children safe, or a concern about potholes on the main street. Groups form, people band together, alliances are forged, and guess what? The concern is usually eradicated.

As I have been thinking, and reading about communities, I came across a wonderful booklet by Mary O'Connell (1988), titled, *The Gift Of Hospitality*. In this work, O'Connell offers an interesting comparison between aspects of community and human services. Her points are important to consider here:

IN ASSISTED SETTINGS	IN THE COMMUNITY
People are known by what's wrong, their condition or label	People are known as individuals
People are incomplete, need to be changed or fixed	People are as they are with opportunity to dream
Relationships are unequal-workers do for the client	Relationships are reciprocal
People are broken into parts, separated into groups	People are accepted as whole and viewed as part of the whole society
Problems are solved by consulting authorities, policy, procedure	People seek answers from their own experience and the wisdom of others
There is no room to acknowledge mistakes and uncertainty	People can make honest efforts and acknowledge honest mistakes and fears
All problems have a rational solution	There is room for confusion, mystery, and recognition that some things are beyond human control

Another analyst of community issues is John McKnight, of Northwestern University. In a provocative article, titled "Regenerating Community," McKnight (1987), also contrasts communities to human services. He shared that:

❖ Human services operate on control
❖ Communities operate on consent

❖ Human services are often slow and deliberate
❖ Communities respond quickly

❖ Human services require solutions go through channels
❖ Communities inspire creative solutions

As I think of McKnight's points, many examples of human services I have visited come to mind. First and foremost is that control in services to people with disabilities is omnipresent. I know group homes where any visitors to the house must sign in. Imagine that the next time you walk into a friend's home.

As for human services being deliberate, I am struck by the barriers staff have often to jump through to get the simplest of things. Every good idea posed must be subjected to a task force to study and then render a decision. The time wasted in this process is amazing. I have a friend who works for Associated

Press. He is often frustrated when he phones as I am usually in some meeting. Each time he teases me, I am reminded of the never ending cascade of task forces, advisory committees, and coalitions that I am part of. I don't know about other fields, but it seems human services have more than their fair share.

As for channels, most human services function through policy and procedure. I once remember getting a phone call from a new staff member who was frantic about a person we support who was missing. After he told me Jim was missing he asked, "What's our policy on missing persons?" You can imagine my answer. I screamed, "Find Jim!!!"

Yet, policies and formalities abound. Every time a new challenge occurs, a new policy is designed to attempt to answer and provide a smooth guideline to solving the problem. We must recognize that this propensity to develop policies and procedures is a direct manifestation of the medical/expert paradigm. They are attempts to predict and standardize actions; an effort to establish formulas.

I also recall a friend who works at a group home in the Midwest. We were talking about wine, and I told him about a great bottle of wine I received as a Christmas gift from a fellow we support. He said to me in amazement, "You can accept gifts from clients?" I responded, "Of course." He then said, "We can't. We have a policy against it." Imagine that. A basic interchange of human expression is perverted because a policy prevents gifts between staff and residents.

Now, let's pause here and ponder this. I'm sure somewhere down the line, the program my friend works for probably had one of their staff take advantage of a resident. As a result, all expression of gifts between people were dictated to stop. Talk about stretching an issue to perversion; we must inspect the reality of our actions.

The examples go on. In my own state of Pennsylvania, a major state office which funds community living arrangements for people with retardation labels, has a policy that all liquid detergent must be locked up in residents' apartments. This happened because a few years ago, quite by mistake, a fellow with retardation drank some Lux liquid and got sick. Now every residential program this department finds in Pennsylvania, which supports thousands of people, has pad locks on the kitchen cabinets. Just like your home, right?

Indeed, once I was appealing for a resident in this same state funded system who was tired of physical therapy and wanted a break. This man, and the eight other folks we support who lived near him in their own apartment have their lives riddled with therapy. During the day, during the evenings, and for some, even on the weekend. Most of these folks have no say in what they get, how the therapy is rendered, or when it happens. I asked an official for some leniency. After all, I pleaded, this is their home. She said, in a scolding fashion, "Oh, but you're wrong. This is not their home, but a program."

This issue of who creates the rules and who has to follow the rules is an important notion to ponder. In a thoughtful article, *Rules: The New Institutions*, Steve Holburn (1990), explores this concept of how programs in the community can be as rigid as any institution. He states:

> . . . when the contingencies of rule following are powerful and rules themselves inaccurate, ineffective rules based behavior will be dominant; in other words, people (staff) will do what they are told, even if it does not work. This phenomena can influence the behavior of therapists, teachers, and even parents.

When I think about Holburn's thesis and my experience in the field, I must agree. Rules, regulations, and structure have come to dominate most state or federally funded programs in America today. Although this continues to keep the residents of these programs harnessed to an institutional reality, an equally damaging consequence is created with the community. All our rhetoric about people becoming equal members of the community is muted by the institutional structure everyone sees.

And so, rules, regulation, policy, procedure, and control abound. Human service, as much as they try to be typical to life, is nothing more than a bureaucracy. This is alien to how communities operate. No wonder communities are speculative about people with disabilities and resist group homes in their neighborhoods as is documented in countless zoning efforts against group homes.

To reverse these trends, demand that we become students of community. For the most part this means becoming conscious and sensitive to the formal and informal aspects of community. We need to look around. Before we explore community, it is important to differentiate between the terms community and neighborhood. Neighborhood is defined in *The Neighborhood Organizers Handbook* (Warren & Warren, 1979) as:

> referring to the social organizations of a population residing in a geographic proximate locale. This includes not only social bonds between members of the designated population, but all bonds that group has to non-neighbors as well.

As we endeavor to understand community, we must make some differentiations. In the book, *Our Community*, Curtis and Mial (1960) suggest five ways to examine communities. These are:

1. As a geographic area
2. As a legal unit of government
3. As a set of attitudes, beliefs, and loyalties

4. As a collection of neighborhoods
5. As a network of associations.

Indeed, community is all of these things, and can be isolated around any particular variable.

Although the term *community* can have broader implications, such as in describing the "disability community," my use for community in this chapter is similar to that of neighborhood. That is, a smaller proximity that relates to walking and relating space between where people live and the goods and services they need to enrich their lives.

FUNCTIONS OF COMMUNITY

In the aforementioned book, *The Neighborhood Organizers Handbook,* by Warren and Warren, six distinct functions of community are identified. A review of these functions offer a start point in this examination of community.

1. *As a sociability arena.* Here they mean the neighbor-to-neighbor chats that occur that are driven by proximity.

2. *As an interpersonal influence center.* This category refers to the advice we get from neighbors when we are in a jam.

3. *Mutual aid.* This level deals with the banding together that occurs during emergencies.

4. *As an organizational base.* Here they refer to the associations that form within community. Most common would be groups such as the PTA.

5. *As a reference group.* This dimension suggests an identification, often associated with pride, or location. Often communities will rally around a successful high school or college sports team.

6. *As a status arena.* This final category serves to allow neighbors to gauge or parade their status in the community. Things like additions to the home or a new car are often measures.

These functions offer us some sense of the purpose that communities serve. All or some of these six functions come into play when people gather together in some common proximity.

∽

People do not live together merely to be together. They live together to do something together.

Ortega Y. Gasset

THE FORMAL DIMENSIONS

Most communities have some formal structure. This is the official governing body that oversees the actions of community. For some entities, this is a mayor. Other communities have commissioners. Some areas have a mayor and a professional town, or borough manager. These positions can be full-time, or part-time. They can be paid, or voluntary positions. Except for town managers, these are usually elective offices. To this extent, these folks are accountable to the public.

Consider your town. What type of system do you have? Do you know your community officials, and where they stand on issues? Are you familiar with the tax base, the percentage you pay to sustain your town government? Are you aware of the services offered in your community? Who would you call, if, say your street needed paved or resurfaced?

Find out these things. Become aware of your community. This is the first step to begin an understanding, and to culture a community that cares about all its citizens. Further, investigate the communities where people you care about live. Look into these same issues. Find out about the formal structure. It's a key stepping stone to participation and interdependence.

Aside from the formal political structure, communities can also be analyzed within a typography. That is, communities do fit categories that can formally or informally influence how the community operates. Again, citing Warren and Warren, six basic community types can be considered. These are:

❖ *Integral* — Here the community is closely linked and woven together. Neighbors have a deep and common bond.

❖ *Parochial* — At this type, the community is bonded together, but some of the close linkages may be missing.

❖ *Diffuse* — This third level finds a community that has a common identity, but missing some of the close interactions.

❖ *Stepping-Stone* — This community type allows for interactions and linkages, but is often missing in identity.

❖ *Transitory* — These communities offer some linkages between neighbors, but are missing the depth of identity.

❖ *Anomic* — This final category finds little commonalty between neighbors. People keep to themselves and have little, if any, reliance on each other.

These community types are helpful in a review of the challenges of interdependence. If we plan to make connections among and between neighbors, or facilitate this occurrence, we need to understand the territory. Quite clearly, the typography identified by Warren and Warren shows a cascading interpersonal dimension of communities. If we were making plans to connect, or even to help people make some selection, having a sense of the community type would be most helpful.

Like any other analysis, however, this typography can have its limitations. Not all communities are so clean cut or predictive. We need to use this list, and any other type of social tool as a guide, and not necessarily gospel.

Indeed, this brief formal analysis of communities helps set up the fun part of understanding communities, a look at their informal nature.

THE INFORMAL DIMENSIONS

Human beings are not like amoebas, we're not things. We're much more like coral, we're interconnected. We cannot survive without each other.

Willard Gaylin

As fascinating as formal systems and politics are, even more intriguing are the informal systems of community. By informal, I am referring to those people and places where the real action happens. These are the diners and barber shops and laundromats. This is where people gather, and where relationships are forged.

Every community has an informal pulse. In my town, it's the Shop-n-Save supermarket. In fact, the Shop-n-Save has become so popular, that they recently expanded their diner section to accommodate more people. On any given Sunday, the best and brightest of town are there. Deals are cut, acquaintances are renewed, and gossip abounds.

When you think about your town's pulse, know that the influential people usually meet there. These are the people who know people and things about your town. They are also the gatekeepers to acceptance and relationships. They are keys to finding places that "tickets" can get punched.

And what about other mainlines to connections. I have found that barber shops, libraries, beauty shops, and the town newspaper are all great places to hunt. Most of the time these folks know what is happening. They are purveyors of information. Get to know them. Find out what is going on.

As I have come to know more about communities there are some key institutions that can help you in your understanding. These places/settings all can offer entrees to vital people within the community. Consider the following:

CHURCHES

Kindness in words creates confidence. Kindness in thinking creates profoundness. Kindness in giving creates love.

Lao-Tzu

The churches — what wonderful places churches are. First, they promote values of acceptance and hospitality. They are about looking out for one another. They are usually places of openness and welcome. All are vital components to interdependence.

Of course not all churches are this way, but most are, and offer a superb starting point for your community actions. Get to know the churches in your area. Meet with the pastor and learn of the church's activities.

In his recent book, *Who Needs God,* Rabbi Harold Kushner (1990) explores the role of the church. Kushner is convinced that a major role, perhaps the most important role, of the church, is to build community. He feels that churches are fulfilling a spot that community once played in harboring people in an act of communality.

Today in communities, churches host festivals and spur on opportunities for people to gather. In many regards, they are a beacon of hospitality to and for people.

As I write these words I am drawn to my own church, Mothers of Sorrows in McKees Rocks, PA. Like most churches, Mothers of Sorrows has ministered for years to the predominantly Italian community that surrounds the parish. Every year, the church is instrumental in conducting community festivals and events that bring the neighbors together in celebration.

One important role that the church has paid special attention to is the ethnic heritage of our community. At the festival of St. Anthony, for example, the community has continued the age-old Italian custom of parading a large baby doll through the streets where people walk along to the sounds of a marching band, complete with accordions and tambourines.

Now, it is not my point to get you to join a church and practice religion. Each of us need to wrestle with the ways and means to personal spirituality for ourselves. It is my point, however, to suggest that churches can serve as a linking point to viable, natural relationships for people who have become distantiated from community.

COMMUNITY SPACE

Every community has open and public space designed for community use. This space may have some specific focus, but by and large it is for the community residents. Some examples of this community space are:

❖ *Centers* — Some neighborhoods have centers specific to informal gatherings. These areas are centers where bingo might be held, community festivals carried out, or general meeting places. Indeed, some developers have found the wisdom of the community centers and have built this concept into the designs of all-purpose communities. I recently was in Buffalo to help some friends explore options for residential supports. We visited an inclusive community that had a community center smack in the middle of the apartments. During our visit the center hosted a library, day care

ᑤ

Segregation is the offspring of an illicit intercourse between injustice and immorality.

M.L. King

center, bulletin board, and huge coffee urn. Folks from the community were sitting around, much like an old-time community square.

❖ *Libraries* — For many communities, the library is often the central gathering place. They, too, often have day care centers, class rooms, and general meeting rooms. Along with serving the role of informational resource, the library has become a key central place for many communities. Although my own community does not have a library, often when I travel, I will seek out the public library and hang out. It is amazing the activity and spirit of communality that can be observed.

❖ *Municipal Buildings* — Other communities use the municipal offices as a point of central gathering. Not only are these buildings places to vote and pay taxes, but they also serve to link people together. A good example of this is found in the towns of New England. With the town meeting spirit of these communities, the municipal buildings do more than just host official business.

❖ *Private Clubs* — Most communities have a variety of private clubs with buildings and office space. Often these entities can serve the same purpose of communality. These include service clubs such as the Lions, Elks, Kiwanas, VFW's and others. Additionally, places such as the Boys' Club or YMCA can serve the same type of purpose.

❖ *Parks/Town Square* — These spaces, usually outdoors, are municipally operated and available as gathering places for informal community business. When you think of town squares, the image of seniors playing chess and children playing hopscotch comes to mind. These are important places of connecting and hospitality.

THE GREAT GOOD PLACES

A few years ago, a friend of mine told me about a book, *The Great Good Places*, by Ray Oldenburg (1988). This book chronicles and describes the gathering places found in most communities. Usually, these are private establishments that have an uncanny ability to offer people a warm sense of hospitality. Some of these are:

❖ *Taverns* — From the time of the first settlers in America, the tavern has served an important role of communality. In most any town in America today, on most every evening, community neighbors can be found sharing a drink and story in the local tavern.

☙

How quickly we build barriers around ourselves, not only to protect our authority but also to give us a certain strength, because we feel weak under the weight of it.

J. Vanier

Indeed, many travellers to new communities will seek out the tavern for a place to feel at home. The popularity of the TV show "Cheers," is a testimony to the popularity and personality of the tavern.

❖ *Diners* — Along with drink, food plays a critical role in hospitality. There is no question about the significance of "breaking bread." Diners play an important role in the establishment of community, by offering a small and personal place for people to gather around food and drink.

❖ *Hardware Stores* — There is something alluring about an old fashioned hardware store. Maybe it's the owner, or manager, who knows almost everything, or the intrigue of the stuff that things are made of. Whatever, hardware stores in some towns serve an important role of being a great, good place.

In my town, we have Ace Hardware. A trip to Ace, and opportunity to talk with Lee, the owner is truly an experience. The first thing you notice upon entering Ace, is the classical music. There is something oxymoronic about classical music and plumbing supplies, but at Ace they seem harmonious. Next, you are struck by the cluttered, and somewhat dirty aisles of stuff. Then there is Lee, a mustachioed wizard who knows everything about anything. I have been going to Lee's hardware store with my dad since I was a kid, and I can never remember leaving the store without the item or gizmo we needed to solve the problem. In more recent years, I have noticed that other community sages hang out at Ace, as well. I guess great minds are attracted to each other.

❖ *Construction Sites* — Much like the lure of a hardware store, is the draw of a good construction site. I now understand why they put peep holes in the barriers that protect the site from the public — so that they can serve as a great, good place. Next time you drive near a construction site on a clear warm day, note the people who have gathered to monitor the progress.

❖ *Shopping Centers* — As our communities become more sprawling, the local "Main Street" has given way to the malls. Yet people need to gather, and so the malls have become the modern day great good places. Malls now serve the community with bulletin boards, community conveniences such as libraries, food courts to take the place of diners, and opportunities for exercising.
During a recent visit to the suburban mall near my community, I was nearly stampeded by a herd of "walkers" getting their exercise while at the mall.

❖ *Super Markets* — A final great, good place of today's community is often found at the local supermarket. These places offer much more than groceries. My local supermarket has a restaurant, video store, bank machine, and postal services all in one building.

Further, you can buy auto supplies, videos, flowers, books, cards and the like, without ever going into the cold. Without question, our Shop'n Save has become a vital community center. This was driven home to me during a recent election when the local politicians had a debate at the Shop'n Save.

COMMUNICATION

A final central point of consideration when attempting to understand community is to examine the communication activity. All communities have communication patterns that are vital to the bonding of citizens. As with all communication, these patterns are both formal and informal. The places we have just reviewed most often host the informal activities, which is face-to-face chatter between citizens. There are, however, formal patterns that are equally powerful, and vital to applying Interdependence to communities. Some of these are:

❖ *Local Newspaper* — Most towns have a local paper that serves as a hub of the formal communication. School news, political issues, social concerns, births and deaths are all important bits of news that the community must have. When I travel, I always attempt to find and read the most local newspaper available. It's amazing the information you can gather.

❖ *Greensheet* — Along with the local newspaper, most communities also have a Greensheet, or Pennysaver available. These newspapers are predominantly want ads and commercial ads germane to the community. These weekly's also have some stories and local information that can tell you much about the community. Of course, the want ads will tell you some very interesting things about the nature of the community, things that are available, or valuable enough for people to solicit.

❖ *Community Bulletins* — Many communities have central bulletin boards that post formal information on activities and services available. These boards are viable spots to find formal communication patterns. Next time you see a community bulletin board, stop to read it, being sure to look deeper than the specific things listed. See if you can learn about the nature of the community.

❖ *Cable TV* — As electronic communication has become more accessible, the local cable TV station is playing the same role as the local newspaper. Vital information is conveyed, as well as interviews, ads, political activities, and in some cases, community college classes. As technology increases, these cable TV stations will become more interactive, allowing viewers to phone, or punch in responses to topics.

❖ *Urban Newspaper* — Many urban newspapers, recognizing the emergence of local communities, have developed suburban inserts for particular sections of the greater metropolitan area. My paper for example, *The Pittsburgh Post Gazette* has a regular Wednesday insert devoted to the particular locality East, West, South or North. This insert is filled with stories, and news specific to that region.

❖ *Church Bulletins* — Most churches and synagogues have weekly bulletins that are made available to their parishioners. These bulletins list out not only church issues, but will focus on community concerns as well. Often Rabbis or Pastors are searching for material for their bulletins.

READING COMMUNITY

As we strive to be more astute about communities, there are many activities and actions to better prepare us. Certainly, there are important points about civics that we should know about government and community structure. Knowing how a community formally operates is vital. To this point there are things we can find to read. Some good references are in the bibliography in this book, but a community library also has excellent resources on community.

Another type of reading we can do, however, is related to the clues evident in any community you might visit. Every time I enter a community, I challenge myself to see how much I can guess about the community, based on what I observe. Although this is not scientific, or supported in the literature, here are some of the things I look for, and what they tell me about the community.

Cars — A very obvious aspect of any community:

❖ Are the cars owned by the residents?
❖ Are there cars on the street, or do people have garages?
❖ If there are cars on the street, how new are they?
❖ Current models, or older vehicles?
❖ How well kept are they?
❖ Are they clean and seemingly in a good state of repair?
❖ Do they have bumper stickers?
❖ If so, what do they say or advertise?

Clues — Certainly, cars can tell us much about the community and their owners. You can tell economic levels and taste of the owners. You can surmise the

Until you have become really, in actual fact, as brother to everyone, brotherhood will not come to pass.

Fyodor Dostoyevski

owner's age and style by the model and color. Clean, or meticulous cars will suggest the owner's interest in detail and pride in their possessions. Vans connote children, trucks suggest commerce and cars point to smaller units of family. Of course, bumper-stickers often show the owner's political or stylistic bent. Advertisements for radio stations, political candidates, environmental concerns, colleges/universities, political issues and the like all show up on the bumpers of peoples' cars.

General Appearance — The overall appearance and state of repair of the community can tell important things. The next time you enter a community, consider the following:

- ❖ How do the houses look? Are they fresh looking and kept well?
- ❖ Are the lawns and shrubs attractive? Are there flowers present?
- ❖ Do the streets have sidewalks and are they walkable?
- ❖ Do trees line the streets?
- ❖ How much space is between the houses or buildings?
- ❖ Are there fences or barriers between where people live?
- ❖ Do the homes have porches, with furniture and signs that people sit out?
- ❖ Are the streets in good shape?
- ❖ Is the residential area linked to commercial areas by bus stops, or neighborhood stores?
- ❖ What is the general appearance of the closest commercial area?
- ❖ Are stores open and attractive?
- ❖ Are there many alleys? If so, do the alleys appear safe, would you walk down them?

Clues — As you might imagine, general appearance demonstrates pride and safety in the community. Sidewalks and porches tell you about the movement and actions of people. Further, external actions suggest that people come in contact with each other on a fairly regular basis. Proximity between houses, or barriers present, such as fences or walls, also points to a communality, or lack of it. Certainly, commercial and civic space such as stores, streets, bus service and the like, all help us get a closer feel for the receptivity of the area.

Billboards — not every area has billboards, but those that do shout out interesting indicators. Usually billboards are on the highways leading to the community. Regardless, look for the following:

❖ Where are the billboards located?
❖ Are they near to the homes?
❖ Are they clustered or sporadically located?
❖ What type of products do they advertise?
❖ What are the themes of the products?
❖ Do you see some trends or consistencies in the ads?
❖ Have any of the billboards, or ads they display been defaced or altered beyond what the advertiser might do?

Clues — It is vital to remember that advertisers are in the business to make money. They do their homework on who buys, or might want to buy their product. To this extent, you can predict that the product advertised is one that the community has been gauged to need or want. Thus, you should pay attention to the products displayed. Bank ads might suggest that potential investors are present. Alcohol, or cigarette ads might reveal something about the residents. Cultural, or civic events can suggest a style and background of the people who live nearby. (Certain ads might suggest certain ethnic groups.) Clustered ads are implosive, and suggest that the residents need to be bombarded. Altered ads might tell us that people in the community are rejecting what the advertiser is selling.

Taverns, Bars, and Diners — These common and public places are mainstays in any community. As you continue your analysis, consider:

❖ Are there many bars, and how close are they to each other?
❖ Do they look inviting?
❖ Are they neighborhood taverns, or are they chains?
❖ Do they attract men and women, or just men?
❖ Are there "regulars" older or younger?
❖ Is the owner known in the community?

Clues — Much of what the answers to these questions tell us is obvious. They are factors of desirability. The more desirable and folksy, the more they add to the community. If the owner is local, there is more of a chance that the bar or tavern is a great good place. Chains suggest a transiency or autonomy of the community.

Pets — The emergence and importance of pets in our society is an interesting trend in and of itself. As you explore community, what do you see and make of the presence of animals?

❖ What kinds of pets and how many do you notice?
❖ Are they, on average, large or small?
❖ Are they chained?
❖ Are residents observed walking their pets?
❖ Do they reside outside (in pet houses) or do they seem to be indoor pets?
❖ How are they treated?

> **Clues** — Pets can demonstrate a community receptivity. People who usually have pets, I have found, are often open to other people. That is, of course, unless their pets are guard dogs designed to keep people away. Indoor pets seem to suggest that the owners have a kindness about them. Larger pets might suggest an aggressiveness or authoritarian slant.

Presence of Children — Children in communities are a vital element in gaining a sense of the community character. Consider the following:

❖ Does the community have children present?
❖ Are there toys in the yards, swing sets, bicycles, and the like present?
❖ Are there parks and civic recreation areas close by?
❖ Is there a little league present of other type of organized sports?
❖ Are there boys/girls clubs, scouts or YMCA/YWCA centers nearby?

> **Clues** — Children suggest a receptivity and patience present in the community. Organized activities show a civic concern and a broader sense of participation on the part of the neighbors. In many regards, happy laughing children indicate a healthy community.

Churches — Spirituality is a key factor in gauging the receptivity of communities. And the way people worship often is a solid case to welcoming and hospitality. Consider these questions:

❖ What is the presence and diversity of churches/synagogues in the area?
❖ Are most denominations represented, or does there seem to be one major order in the community?
❖ Are the churches large in size and congregation, or smaller?
❖ Do they have a school attached, offer Sunday School.

❖ Do they have a marque that announces the sermon and thrust of the worship?

Clues — Churches, of course, offer thoughts on the spirituality of the community. They can tell you some things about the ethnic flavor of the neighborhood. They can also show community economics as the welfare of the church is tied directly to its parishioners. Schools and Sunday School reveal a commitment to the future of the congregation and spirituality in the community.

Events - These general gatherings are important to any community. As you analyze your community, consider the following:

❖ As you explore the community do you see evidence of community celebrations?
❖ Are there festivals, parades, carnivals, and other types of organized events that occur on a regular basis?
❖ Do people support these events both in participation, or observation?
❖ Does the community seem to be proud of the event by advertising?

Clues — Events tell you some things about the organization, pride, and history of the community. They suggest that the community leaders, elected and appointed, are working to make, or keep, their community viable. Celebrations and laughter also show a happiness and willingness to commune with one another. These are signs of community health and vitality.

Recognize that this "reading" of community is not suggested as a know-all or be-all. Rather, it offers some clues and cues that might help you to get started in understanding communities. It suggested some "feel" for the community and can offer a real hope in the reunion of the disenfranchised person. It can also give us a sense of ways and means that the person can practice interdependence. That is, some of the items just reviewed can serve as places for people to get "tickets" punched.

Another important reason for the review is to prompt any person reading this book to consider these items in your own community. Clearly the concept of interdependence in community starts with you and me.

We need to understand that the basic elements of this book are not designed as a cookbook to "apply" to people who are disenfranchised, but to turn inward, toward ourselves. All of us are members of some community. How hospitable and open is your own community? More importantly, what are you doing to make your community more welcoming of people who have some difference about them?

Without question there is much we all need to know about community. The items reviewed in this chapter are merely a scratch of the surface. There is further reading, writing and study to do.

We know that people who are different want to belong to community. We also know that the agencies we have developed to do this for people with difference are not working well. Further, these very agencies may be damaging the efforts of reunion, because they continue to prompt what is wrong with people, and usually keep the apart from community. Lastly, the very goal of the entire effort, community reentry, is a field that most people associated with those who are disenfranchised know little about. This chapter has been an introduction, a mere prick of the consciousness, about the focal point of the real goal — community interdependence.

=================

Belonging, not escape,
is the imperative moral value.

R.A. Nisbet

6

Conclusion

*Satisfaction lies in the effort,
not in the attainment.
Full effort is full victory.*

Mohandas Gandhi

6

Conclusion

Often, when I am asked to do a talk on interdependence or empowerment, I use slides to complement the presentations. My slides are either key points or concepts, graphics, or photos. As you may have surmised by now, a lot of my slides are also of quotes to drive home points or create a segway to a new concept.

I conclude most of my presentations, however, with a slide of my children, Dante, Gianna, and Santino. As I flash this last picture, it allows me the opportunity to mention my children, how much they mean to me, and how much I miss them as I travel. It also allows me to introduce the final point about interdependence; that of the future.

When I show my family slide, it reminds me how essential and self-serving the concept of interdependence is for now and future generations. It also allows me an opportunity to escape the "white knight for the disabled" image that people might conjure up from my talks.

Quite simply, with interdependence there are four concluding themes:

1. Under our prevailing paradigms, people who have some difference are usually subject to being perceived and treated in a devalued way. This devaluation leads to direct or indirect separation from community.

2. Any one of us, at any time, is at risk of being injured, getting sick, becoming poor, growing old, or becoming otherwise different and then devalued. All of us are vulnerable.

3. Interdependence offers an alternative that balances the equation, and keeps people connected to community. It provides a backdrop of relationships in an effort to retain a sense of community.

4. Finally, a diversity in community enriches life for all of us. By having a multiplicity of varied people, all who are welcomed and respected adds a flavoring to community that is irreplaceable.

So, as I show my children at the end of my talks, I can equate interdependence for all of us. That is, interdependence, although discussed in this book in conjunction with disability issues, is not really about disability at all. Rather, it is about people and society. It is about community. It is about harmony. Indeed, it is about the future.

This notion of harmony is an interesting one. In music, we know that two different notes, when put together create a blend that is richer than the two single notes. Indeed when you add a third or fourth note, the result is a powerful sound that hangs together.

Recently, I have become much more aware of musical harmony. My daughter, Gianna, has been studying the piano, and as we sit to review her lessons I am struck by the brilliance of chords. When we play a typical three note chord, a C-E-G for example, the sound is warm. Then when we get creative and add a B, the sound intensifies. If we shift the fourth note from a B to B flat, the sound is very different — just with one half step. What beauty, creativity and mood is set by stringing these notes together.

The same results of beauty, creativity, and mood are found, I believe, in community when we string together three or four different people. As with our piano, the sound enriches and intensifies.

This harmonious blend of people shows its depth when we consider groups. Consider, for example, your team at work, or if you don't work any other type of small group you belong to. Once the unique contributions of the team are known, understood and appreciated a certain harmony is formed.

Now, think back to that same group and when the constellation may have changed — a new member added, or someone might have gone. The addition or deletion of a member, much as with a note added or deleted from a musical chord, probably changed the reality of the group.

A few years ago, a friend of mine from Vancouver, B.C. sent me a wonderful book, *Gifts of the Lotus* (Hanson, 1974). This little pocketbook of spiritual thoughts is divided into 12 chapters, each associated with a month and character theme such as "freedom, truth, courage, humility, etc." Each chapter has 30 short thoughts associated with the character theme. As you might suspect, there is a chapter devoted to harmony. As we continue to reflect on this concept of harmony, let me share here, a few of the thoughts on harmony:

❖ Harmony is unity in diversity.
❖ ...the very heart of nature is harmony, the very fabric and structure of the universe is coordination and cooperation, spiritual union.
❖ Beauty of style and harmony and grace and good rhythm depend on simplicity.
❖ Wherever life is there is the process of building; different elements are brought together into relations which make of them a living whole, capable of functioning together in harmony.

There is more on harmony in *Gifts of the Lotus*, but these make the point. Harmony is a goal of interdependence. We need to think about it and strive to reach it.

Earlier in this work, I used a quote from Martin Luther King that focused on the interconnectedness of life. King said, "I can't be what I ought to be, and you can't be what you ought to be, until I am what I ought to be." This theme underscores another concluding aspect of interdependence, that our growth and welfare is interconnected.

If you think about life in your community, you are bonded through a similarity of locale, shops, churches, school district, and other common space, yet through the diversity of your neighbors and community, you are inspired to grow and develop. In allowing each person to be welcomed and accepted, all people grow.

To this extent, interdependence is vital to all, not just people who are disenfranchised. Our welfare is vested in each of us, and the interdependent paradigm attempts to offer a backdrop to make this happen.

And so, when I end talks or discussions about interdependence, I relate future thoughts and actions to my family. In fact, my extended family offers an interesting lens in which to understand interdependence. As I mentioned, the Condeluci family, (at least 15 families of us) live up on a family compound in a small industrial town, McKees Rocks, about seven miles from downtown Pittsburgh, PA. We've been on or near our "hill" since 1918, now pushing our fifth generation. My children play on the same street and fields that my dad, now 75, did as a child.

In our years on "Condeluci Hill", we have built a pool and nearby meeting hall, affectionately called "La Stanza". This center serves as a focal point for family gatherings and functions. The walls are adorned with five generations of Condeluci pictures and memorabilia. We now have some 125 Condeluci relatives who at some point or another during the year, make a gathering at La Stanza.

Indeed, every night (except when temperatures dip into the single digits) the family elders gather at La Stanza for coffee, Italian pastries, and good conversations. A little less frequently, though more than you can imagine, we children and grandchildren gather too, and listen to the stories.

I built my home on Condeluci Hill in 1976; across the street from my mom and dad, and directly beside my sister, Jan. I was the 12th home added to the compound. We have since added three more of my cousins.

When I tell people about our homestead, or invite people to my home, I get some interesting reactions. Most people cannot relate to this type of family intensity. Many ask how we can handle being so close to parents and relatives. People assume we have no privacy. Some people wonder how much we fight, or if we have serious spats. Other people tell me they could never live so close to their relatives.

Now, all of these reactions amaze me. Imagine a society where being close to family is considered abhorrent; where wanting to exchange stories and to celebrate with each other is taken as being different. At times, I'm sure some people take my family situation as "cute" or "quaint," but not with real seriousness. It is as if we are time warped from an ancient generation; or living a Walton Mountain family.

Regardless of personal responses, however, people who hear the story of "Condeluci Hill" react with warmth and, to a degree, loss. It's as if the intensity of my family interactions hit a nerve for them. Their reactions suggest a wish they could be closer to family. The story of "Condeluci Hill" breaks the crust off the family patterns that exist for them and calls forth patterns they wish could be.

In reality, my family, and life on "Condeluci Hill" is a strong example of interdependence. The bond of family keeps us strongly connected, yet all 15 families have grown in diverse and unique ways. We come together regularly as a "community," but when we do, the exposure we offer that is different, promotes a growth.

Indeed, I feel secure in exploring the unique perspectives of a family member even when I might strongly disagree. The security of our community allows me the space and safety to challenge and grow. I always know that, regardless of my perspective, I will be accepted. This is a powerful notion of security.

This phenomena, when you think of it, has a wonderful cycle to it. That is, the more I am free to think and challenge, the more I respect and work to understand the perspective of the person with whom I disagree. Rather than polarize around issues, which in fact leads to no real growth, this freedom leads to newer visions of understanding.

This approach is really not new. In fact, colleges and universities have attempted to create interdependent environments for a long time. The true university atmosphere is intended to be a place where people can think, differ, compare, and dialogue about concepts and themes of community interest. The notion is that students are free to discover, and in this freedom, respect for difference will grow.

Today, however, there is a growing debate about this agenda and the reality of the universities. Some suggest that the openness necessary in this type of discovery is being undermined. Alan Bloom's (1989) hugely successful book, *The Closing of the American Mind*, examines the variables that have contributed to the decay of scholarly activity.

More recently, debate that has affected openness remains an effort to promote a "politically correct" campus atmosphere. Although this agenda suggests a politically balanced approach to diverse people, primarily through language and access, some argue that this effort is closing off an openness of expression. Some feel that the "PC agenda" (as it is called), goes too far in promoting its ideals that it is a sort of tyrannical form of McCarthyism.

These critics suggest that the intimidation of those who promote a politically correct campus, in effect stifle some types of freedom of expression. On the other hand, those supporting PC feel that oppressive and demeaning ways of referring to people and groups is the real form of intimidation.

Regardless of this debate, any time that external fear or pressure promotes an agenda, the natural elements of Interdependence will be affected. If either party is not comfortable in atmosphere, the elements of acceptance will be perverted or worse, eliminated.

In the aforementioned report, *Toward A State of Esteem*, prepared by the California Task Force (1990), to promote self esteem, this issue of acceptance and growth is acknowledged. It states:

> We cannot give high self-esteem to anyone, but we can help create an affirming environment in which people can more realistically choose to esteem themselves. Doing so also represents our taking personal responsibility for living our commitment, putting it into action in our daily lives and relationships.

The same is true in the wider communities of which we are all a part - neighborhoods, schools, workplaces, professional societies, and social service, political and religious groups. When we act on the conviction that all human beings, including ourselves, deserve to be treated with dignity and respect, we create a new environment of health and growth and community.

There is a strong lesson in thinking about acceptance and security as a stepping stone to growth. The more we can promote the points of our similarity as members of community, the more we can set the stage for the acceptance of difference. This acceptance of difference leads to a respect that can prompt our own growth.

On "Condeluci Hill," as with any other accepting community, there is a hospitality to any of our political or ideological differences. This hospitality is a vital ticket to change and growth. In fact, when challenged in an opinion in a family discussion, I am driven to research both sides of the dispute. This offers a much more focused opportunity for me to make my point.

In *Life 101*, Roger and McWilliams (1990) take a look at this issue of acceptance. Although they focus on basic personal acceptance their thoughts are germane to a review of community acceptance, much like we have on "Condeluci Hill." They state:

Acceptance is not a state of passivity or inaction. We are not saying you can't change the world, right wrongs or replace evil with good. Acceptance is, in fact, the first step to successful action.

If you don't fully accept a situation precisely the way it is, you will have difficulty changing it. Moreover, if you don't fully accept the situation, you will never really know if the situation should be changed.

When you accept, you relax; you let you become patient. This is an enjoyable (and effective) place for their participation or departure...

When you're in a state of nonacceptance, it's difficult to learn. A clenched fist cannot receive a gift, and a clenched psyche - grasped tightly against the reality of what must not be accepted - cannot easily receive a lesson.

To this point, an environment that is basically welcoming, one that sees the similarity of people, is the essential starting point of interdependence. Once this base is set, we are then comfortable enough to be challenged and stretched to grow and develop.

To reach this level of inclusion in our society, however, will not come that easily. Years and years of the crust of exclusionary paradigms have set their course. To this challenge of inclusion, Jack Pearpoint (1990), of the Centre for Integrated Education and Community in Toronto, Canada, stated in a paper (1990):

> *My analysis identifies two opposing trends, two waging factions - inclusion versus exclusion... The debate is between people who believe in exclusivity, and those who believe in inclusion.*
>
> *I believe that inclusive options (all welcome) will utilize the talents of people who would be discarded and written off in the exclusive model. The "outsiders" will bring new perspective and new talents to policy conundrums where we are in a rut and need "fresh ideas."*

The unstated underlying assumptions (for exclusion) are, among others, that:

❖ We are not all equal in capacity or value.
❖ It is not feasible to give equal opportunity.
❖ We must choose – thus train an elite who will take care of the "rest."
❖ They will benefit through the trickle-down theory.

Inclusion is the opposite and works from opposite assumptions:

❖ We are all equal in value; however, each has unique capacities.
❖ All people can learn.
❖ All people have contributions to make.
❖ We have a responsibility and an opportunity to give every person the chance to make a contribution.
❖ The criterion for inclusion is breathing - not IQ, income, color, race, sex or language.

We all have the power to listen to "voices" that are seldom heard. If we choose to make the time, to learn to listen, and to struggle with the pain and frustration that disempowered people feel, we will see new visions, feel new energy, and find hope in our future. There is a power in the powerless. We can be catalysts, or encrusted residue. The choice is ours.

This book has been an effort to make the theoretical justification for the real action that must happen in community. Knowing and accepting the basics of paradigms is the foundation for making interdependence happen. This has been the goal and intent of this book.

Clearly however, there are future books, articles, writings, and stories that must come forth to help us actualize interdependence. Further exploration and dialogue must occur in this area. As you might imagine, I have some thoughts and ideas here, but that is grist for another book at another time.

For now, it is important for us to think and talk about interdependence; to study and debate its focus and place in rehabilitation. As I have pointed out in various sections of this work, my traditional colleagues and friends in the field are not sure what to make of this message and my presence. Clearly, they know that people with disabilities (or other type of disenfranchisement), their families, advocates, and students of community are all engaged by the message. There is a basic chord that is struck — we all can feel it and relate to the idea of change. They also know that the traditional approaches, by and large, are not working.

Yet, their paradigmatic roots are so deep that they have a basic problem with interdependence. Some say it is too simple or easy a concept to have real credence. Others feel that it expects too much from the community or from the person with disabilities — that the problems of disenfranchisement are so complex that the community cannot handle them.

As I conclude this book, I feel that some of these critiques have been addressed. The body of this text speaks for itself, and some people will always have problems. You remember Lincoln's advice about pleasing all the people all the time.

In fact, I did not really write this book for the professionals, although I was encouraged and prompted by hundreds. I wrote this book more for myself, as an effort to harness something I have seen and feel is necessary, for rehabilitation and for the community. I also wrote the book for the many people, from all corners of disenfranchisement, who have felt the same frustration and struggles I have.

As I close this book, the holidays have just concluded and we are entering a brand new year. Like all other new years before and to follow, it is a time of reflection and anticipation. In the media around us, we are swamped with sight and experiences of the past year, the ups and the downs. These are gauges that help us measure how we have done; the things that have worked and those that have not.

In the new year, we are also confronted with baited anticipation; predictions, hopes and aspirations. People make resolutions, and we all reflect on how we need to be better, more caring people and society. We pledge that we will take advantage of opportunities to help out and be more sensitive.

It is appropriate that I be concluding this work at the year's end. I have worked on it most of the year, trying to put it to bed as the holidays near, not being satisfied, wishing I could be more expressive and a better writer. Aside from these typical writer's hesitancies, however, I have a broader sense of reflection. It's as if the end of the year is an interesting metaphor for rehabilitation in general.

Looking back over the shoulder, there are many things that human services have done well and that have worked. The rehabilitation of Howard Rusk and Mary Switzer has been successful at setting the stage and heightening an understanding. Closer to the end of the year, however, we have been struggling. We have not had as many successes; the challenges have grown; things have changed. If Rusk and Switzer were with us today, I believe they would be asking questions about this reality; questioning the paradigm. We must move forward.

Looking ahead, though, is paradoxical. It is easy, as with new year's resolutions, to face the future square in the face and state your plans to change. Doing it is another.

In a way, *Interdependence* is a blueprint for change. It offers a sort of map to what is, and what might be. Like most maps, it can be somewhat complex and confusing. Some directions may be better, or more efficient than others. But, if we are serious about the need to change, as we often are with resolutions, then we should study this map. It can offer a new alternative.

And so, let's put this book down now, and move forward to put some new ideas to work. Around the United States and Canada things are changing and new solutions are necessary. In a number of places, programs and services that utilize an interdependent perspective are in place, but on a whole they are few and far between. More are needed. Let's just do it!

Epilogue

Epilogue

As I put the final elements of the second edition of *Interdependence* to bed, I am more encouraged than ever about the state of service and opportunities for people with disabilities. In my travels and conversations with people around North America, I am constantly impressed by the ideas and actions occurring. More than ever before, people with disabilities are speaking for themselves, and becoming viable members of our culture. I hope in all this forward progress, the concept of *Interdependence* has helped. Yet, I believe there is still so much more work to do; and time is marching on.

As you might imagine, I have more to say about these newer challenges we face in actualizing interdependence. Indeed, as I was called to answer the question, "How do we do interdependence?" I have begun to frame my thoughts toward an inward plane. That is, for interdependence to happen as a concept, we must look at those characteristics that lead to a propensity to include and welcome people. These characteristics, my friends, are not found in technical skills and approaches, but in our spiritual relationships with others. To this extent, then, we must cull out those variables that will allow us, as citizens, to get beyond our differences and find our common humanity.

This task of getting beyond difference and seeing commonality is not an easy one. We are so accustomed to thinking scientifically and analyzing all elements. Most of us have been trained in a secular way, as Newtonian scientists. This Newtonian approach causes us to think in a linear fashion where we process information in a cause and effect way. That is, if someone is not functioning the way we feel they should, then there is some logical cause that must be identified and be replaced or fixed. This scientific structure then causes us to use a medical or expert model to address the problems. In a Newtonians perspective, the person with the disability is the problem. Of course, as you now realize after reading *Interdependence*, people with disabilities are not the problem.

To get beyond seeing difference as the problem, we must push beyond Newtonian science. I am convinced the quantum and chaos theories offer us a far better starting point to think about relationships. Rather than a linear approach, quantum theory suggests a radiant phenomena that considers the whole person and relationships around them. In a forward thinking book, *Leadership and the New Science*, Wheatley (1992), outlines how managers of people can do so much better in their roles if they consider quantum theory. We are not linear creatures, and Wheatley suggests ways we can improve relationships by understanding how entities interact.

In reading, talking, listening, and reflecting, I have just concluded the follow-up to *Interdependence*, that examines the inward question. I have titled this work *Beyond Difference*, and it offers further reflections on culture, difference, and more importantly, variables that can get us beyond difference. If you have found Interdependence to be engaging, I am sure that you will be pleased with *Beyond Difference*.

As I finish this epilogue, I am inclined to use it as epilogues are designed; to update the reader on how things have changed or progressed. For me, things are going well. I am still traveling more than I should, but in a paradoxical way, the travel cuts both ways. When I am away, I miss my family and feel impatient about not nurturing interdependence enough within my organization. Yet, as I travel, I meet fantastic people, learn new things, and get continued motivation to come back home to write more and try new things in my work. It's a creative tension that works for me.

Things on "Condeluci Hill" continue to roll on. The cycle of life pushes us to sadness in funerals and jubilation in new births. These are the poles that lets us know we are alive and feeling. And closer to home, Liz and I have finally given in to the children's pressure and have just bought a dog. Once Santino was lobbied into Dante and Gianna's side, Liz and I were outvoted. So now we have Ziggy, a pure white Bichon with bright eyes and an energetic disposition. If only we could get her housebroken.

At UCP, we continue to evolve and try new things. I am now looking at corporate restructure as a way to organize our continued shift from a traditional model to interdependence. We have repositioned our public identity from UCP to *The Centre for Personal Development*. In this shift, we have begun to maximize our relationship with the community by conducting a variety of events that help build the fabric of the community.

And so, things move on. The days continue to race by and things are changing. There are always new things to do and successes to celebrate. So thanks for deciding to read this book and to take it to this final point. I hope it was helpful and that it has offered some anchor for change. And now I have to shut down this computer and get Ziggy outside. You see, we've got an interdependent thing going.

Bibliography

Bibliography

REFERENCES AND RECOMMENDED READING

Adams, F. (1975). *Unearthing seeds of fire: The idea of Highlander.*
   Winston-Salem, NC: John F. Blair.
Alinsky, S. (1946). *Reveille for radicals*, New York: Random House.
Alinsky, S. (1969). *Rules for radicals*, New York: Random House.
Axelrod, R. (1984). *The evolution of cooperation*, New York: Basic Books.
Banja, J. (1990). Rehabilitation and empowerment, *Archives of Physical
   Medicine and Rehabilitation* Vol. 71.
Barker, J. (1985). *Discovering the future*, Minnesota, IL Press.
Bellah, R., Madsen, R., Sullivan, W., Swidler, A., & Tipton, S. (1985).
   Habits of the heart. New York: Harper and Row.
Bellamy, G. T. (1988). *Supported employment: A community
   implementation guide.* Baltimore: Paul H. Brookes Publishing
   Company.
Bellamy, T., Rhodes, L., Mark, D., & Albin, J. (1988). *Supported
   employment.* Baltimore: Paul H. Brookes Publishing Company.
Biklen, D., & Bogdan, R. (1978). Media portrayals of disabled people: A
   study in stereotypes. *The Bulletin* Vol. 8 - No. 6 & 7.
Biklen, D., & Knoll, J. (1987). The Disabled Minority. In S. Taylor, D.
   Biklen, & J. Knoll (Eds.), *Community integration for people with severe
   disabilities.* New York: Teachers College Press.

213

Blatt, B. (1981). *In and out of mental retardation.* Baltimore: University Park Press.

Bloom, A. (1989). *The closing of the American mnd.* New York: Simon & Schuster.

Bogdan, R., & Biklen, D. (1975) Handicappism. *Social Policy.* Vol. 3, No. 1.

Bowe, F. (1978). *Handicapping America.* New York: Harper & Row.

Bowe, F. (1980). *Rehabilitating America.* New York: Harper & Row.

Bradley, V., & Bersani, H. (1990) *Quality assurance for individuals with developmental disabilities.* Baltimore: Paul H. Brookes Publishing Company.

Branch, T. (1989). *Parting the waters.* New York: Simon & Schuster.

Bronowski, J. (1973). *The ascent of man.* Boston: Little Brown & Co.

Brooks, N. (Ed.) (1984). *Closed head injury: Psychological, social and family consequences.* Oxford: Oxford University Press.

California Task Force to Promote Self-Esteem and Personal and Social Responsibility (1990). *Toward a state of esteem.* Sacramento.

Condeluci, A. (1990). Community factors and successful work Re-entry. In P. Wehman & J. Kreutzer (Eds.), *Vocational rehabilitation for persons with traumatic brain injury.* Baltimore, MD: Aspen Press.

Condeluci, A. (1989). Empowering people with cerebral palsy. *Journal of Rehabilitation* V. 55 No. 2.

Condeluci, A. (1988). *Community residential supports for persons with head injuries.* Washington, DC: United Cerebral Palsy Association.

Condeluci, A., Cooperman, S., & Sief, B. (1987). Independent living: Setting and supports. In M. Ylvisaker & E. Gobble (Eds.), *Community re-entry for head injured adults.* Boston: College Hill Press.

Condeluci, A., Fawber, H., & Gretz-Lasky, S. (1986). A national survey: The need for long-term independent living/vocational rehabilitation services. *NHIF Newsletter*, 5(4).

Condeluci, A., Milton, S., Ingalls, C., & Fenney, M. (1990). Consciousness Quiz from the *Workshop Controversy in the Community.* New Orleans: National Head Injury Foundation Annual Conference.

Condeluci, A., & Swales, P. (1990). *From no one to domeone.* Buffalo: Headway for the Brain Injured.

Conti, G., & Felling, R. (1986). Myles Horton: Ideas that have withstood the test of time. *Adult Literacy and Basic Education.* Vol. 10, No. 1.

Covey, S. (1989) *The 7 habits of highly efective people.* New York: Simon & Schuster.

Crew, N., & Zolla, I. (1983) *Independent lving for physically disabled.* San Francisco: Jossey Bass.

DeJong, G. (1978). Independent living: From social movement to analytical paradigm. *Archives of Physical Medicine and Rehabilitation*, Vol. 60.

DeJong, G. (1983). Defining and Implementing the Independent Living Concept. In N. Crew & I. Zolla (Eds.), *Independent living for physically disabled people.* San Francisco: Josey Bass.

deTocqueville, A. (1883). *Democracy in America.* Edited by J. P. Mayer. Harper & Row, 1966.

Duncan, B., Woods, D. (Eds.) (1989). *Ethical issues in disability and rehabilitation.* New York: World Institute on Disability - World Rehabilitation Fund.

Dunst, C. J., Trivete, C. M., & Deal, A. G. (1988). *Enabling and empowering families.* Cambridge, MA: Brookline Books.

Everson, J., & Moon, M. S., (1987). Transition services for young adults with severe disabilities: Defining professional and parental roles and responsibilities. *J.A.S.H.* Vol. 12, No. 2.

Ferguson, M. (1980). *The aquarian conspiracy.* New York: Tarcher Press.

Forest, M., & Flynn, G. (1988) *With a little help from my friend.* Toronto: Centre for Integrated Education and Community.

Freire, P. (1973). *Education for critical consciousness.* New York: Continuum Press.

Freire, P. (1989). *Pedagogy of the oppressed.* New York: Continuum.

Garret, J., Levine, E. (1973). *Rehabilitation Practices with the Physically Disabled.* New York: Columbia University Press.

Gatto, J. (1989). *Why schools don't educate. The Utney Review.* Summer 1990.

Gaventa, J. (1980). *Power and powerlessness.* Chicago: University of Illinois Press.

Gaventa, J. (1989). *Participatory research in North America: An approach to education presented through a collection of writings.* New Market, TN: Highlander Research and Education Center.

Glenn, M. B., & Rosenthal, M. (1985). Rehabilitation following severe traumatic brain injury. *Seminars in Neurology,* Vol. 5.

Goffman, E. (1961). *Asylums.* New York: Anchor.

Goffman, E. (1963). *Stigma.* New Jersey: Prentice-Hall.

Gold, M. W. (1973). Vocational rehabilitation for the mentally retarded. In N. R. Ellis (Ed.), *International review of research in mental retardation,* 6. New York: Academic Press.

Gold, M. W., & Ryan, K. (1980). Vocational training of mentally retarded. In M. W. Gold (Ed.), *Did I say that? Articles and commentary on the try another way system.* Champaign, IL: Research Press.

Goldenson, R. (1978). *Disability and rehabilitation handbook.* New York: McGraw-Hill.

Goldmann, K., & Sjostedt, G. (1979). *Power, capabilities, interdependence.* London: Sage Publications.

Griffin, J. (1960). *Black like me.* Boston: Houghton-Mifflin.

Gutierrez, L. (1989). Working with women of color: An empowerment perspective. *Social Work.* March Issue.

Hahn, H. (1985). Toward a politics of disability: Definitions, disciplines, and policies. *Social Science Journal* v. 22, No. 4, p. 82-104.

Hampton, H., & Fayer, S. (1990). *Voices of freedom.* New York: Bantam.

Harmon, W. (1970). *An incomplete guide to the future.* New York: Norton Press.

Harris, L. & Associates. (1986). *Disabled Americans self perceptions: Bringing disabled Americans into the mainstream.* Senate Subcommittee on Handicapped Reauthorization Hearing.

Harro, R. (1980). *Social issues training project.* School of Education. University of Mass. Amherst, MA.

Hawson, V. (Ed.) (1974). *Gifts of the lotus.* Wheaton, IL: Theosophical Publishing House.

Holburn, S. (1990). Rules: The new institutions. *Mental Retardation.* Vol 28, No. 2.

Horton, M. (1989). A people's movement to liberate education in *an approach to education presented through a collection of writings.* New Market, TN. Highlander Research and Education Center.

Horton, M. (1990) *The long haul.* New York: Doubleday.

Horton, M., & Freire, P. (1990). *We make the road by walking.* Philadelphia, PA: Temple University Press.

Huenfeld, J. (1970). *The community activist's handbook*. Boston: Beacon Press.

Humphrey, H. (1964). *Integration vs. degregation*. New York: Thomas Y. Crowell Co.

Hutchins, M. P., Renzaglia, A., Stahlman, J., & Cullen, M. E. (1986). *Developing a vocational curriculum for students with moderate and severe handicaps*. Charlottesville, VA: University of Virginia.

Illich, I. (1976). *Medical nemesis*. New York: Pantheon.

Jacobs, H. (1985). The Los Angeles head injury survey: Project rationale and design implications. *The Journal of Head Trauma Rehabilitation*, 2(3).

Jacobs, H. (1987). *Adult community integration*. A paper presented to the National Invitational Conference on Traumatic Brain Injury. Tysons Corners, VA.

Jackman, M. (1983). Enabling the disabled: Perspectives. *The Civil Rights Quarterly* Vol. 15.

Keiffer, C. (1984). "Citizen Empowerment: A Developmental Perspective". *Prevention in Human Services*. 4:2.

Kennedy, W. (1981). Highlander praxis: Learning with Myles Horton. *Teachers College Record*. Vol. 83, No. a.

Knoll, J.,& Ford, A. (1987). Beyond caregiving: A reconceptualization of the role of the residential service provider. In S. Taylor, D. Biklen, & J. Knoll (Eds.), *Community integration for people with severe disabilities*. New York: Teachers College Press.

Kubler-Ross, E. (1975). *On death and dying*. New York: MacMillan.

Kuhn, T. (1962). *The structure of scientific revolution*. Chicago: University of Chicago Press.

Kushner, H. (1990). *Who needs God?* New York. Summit Books.

Kushner, H. (1979) *When bad things happen to good people*. New York, Schocken Books.

Lapon, L. (1986). *Mass murderers in white coats*. Springfield, MA: Research Institute.

Levin, H. S., Benton, A. L.,& Grossman, R. C. (1982). *Neurobehavioral vonsequences of vlosed head injury*. New York: Oxford University Press

Lord, J., & Farlow, D. M. (1990). A dtudy of personal empowerment: Implications for health promotion. *Health Promotion*, Fall Issue.

Lusthaus, E. Euthanasia of persons with severe handicaps: Refuting the rationalizations. *J.A.S.H.* Vol 10, No. 2.

Mahoney, C., Estes, C., & Heumann, J. (1986). *Toward a unified agenda*. Berkeley, CA: World Institute on Disability.

Matheson, J. M. (1982). The vocational outcome of rehabilitation in 50 consecutive patients with severe head injuries. In J. F. Garrett (Ed.), *Austrailian approaches to rehabilitation in Neurotrauma and spinal cord injury*. New York: World Rehabilitation Fund.

McConnell, L. R., & Minston, E. B. (1985). *If...the future of VR*. Morgantown, WV: West Virginia University Research and Training Center.

McCue, M. (1988). *Cognitive, behavioral and vocational rehabilitation of persons with traumatic head injury*. A presentation to the Annual Conference on Cognitive Rehabilitation, Williamsburg, VA.

McKnight, J. (1988). *Beyond community services*. Evanston, IL: Center for Urban Affairs and Policy Research.

McKnight, J. (1987). Regenerating communities. *Social Policy*, Winter Issue.

McKnight, J. (1989). *Do no harm: A policymakers guide to evaluating human services and their alternatives.* Evanston, IL: Center for Urban Affairs and Policy Research.

Merton, R. (1957). *Social theory and social structure.* New York: Free Press.

Mial, D. (1960). *Our community.* New York: New York University Press.

Mount, B., Beeman, P., & Ducharme, G. (1988). *What we are learning about bridge-building.* Manchester, CT: Communities, Inc.

Mount, B., & Zwernik, K. (1987). *It's never too early, It's never too late.* St. Paul, MN: Metropolitan Council.

Mount, B., Beeman, P., & Ducharme, G. (1988) *What are we learning about circles of support.* New Haven: Graphic Futures.

Moyers, W. (1989). *A world of ideas.* New York: Doubleday.

NHIF Directory of Services. (1987). Southborough, MA: NHIF.

Nisbet, J., & Callahan, M. (1987). Achieving success in integrated work settings. In S. Taylor, D. Biklen, & J. Knoll (Eds.), *Community integration for people with severe disabilities.* New York: Teachers College Press.

Nisbit, R. (1972). *Quest for community.* New York: Oxford University Press.

O'Brien, J. (1986). *Discovering community.* Atlanta: Responsive Systems Associates.

O'Brien, J., & Lyle, C. (1987). *Framework for accomplishment.* Decatur, GA: Responsive Systems Associates.

O'Connell, M. (1988). *The gift of hospitality.* Evanston, IL: Center for Urban Affairs and Policy Research.

Oldenburg, R. (1988). *The great good place.* New York: Paragon Press.

Oldendorf, S. (1987). Democratic empowerment and the South Carolina Sea Island citizenship schools: Implications for Appalachian schools, in *An approach to education presented through a collection of writings.* New Market, TN: Highlander Research and Education Center.

Parsons, T. (1951). *Social systems.* Glencoe, IL: Free Press.

Parsons, T. (1964). *Social structure and personality.* New York: Free Press.

Peters, J., & Bell, B. (1986) Horton of Highlander. In P. Jarvis, (Ed.) *Twentieth-century thinkers about adult education.* London: Croom-Helm.

Pearpoint, J. (1990). Inclusion vs. exclusion. *International Review of Education.* UNESCO.

Ploof, D., & Spruill, L. (1990). *Oppression and disability workshop.* Conducted in Pittsburgh, PA. Sponsored by the Commonwealth Institute, Harrisburg, PA.

Prigatano, G. (1989). Work, love, and play after brain injury. *Bulletin of Menninger Clinic,* Vol. 53, No. 5.

Rajecki, D. W. (1982). *Attitudes: Themes and advances.* Sunderland, MA: Sinaver Associates.

Rappaport, J. (1985). The power of empowerment language. *Social Policy* 17(2).

Reed, D. (1981). *Education for a peoples' movement.* Boston: South End Press.

Reich, C. A. (1970). *The greening of America.* New York: Random House.

Roger, J., & McWilliams, P. (1990). *Life 101.* Los Angeles, CA: Prehode Press.

Rusch, F. (1979). Toward the validation of social/vocational survival skills. *Mental Retardation,* 33(2).

Russell, B. (1938). *Power: A new social analysis.* New York: W. W. Norton & Co.

Sacks, O. (1989). *Seeing voices.* Berkeley, CA: University of California Press.

Saranson, S. (1972). *The creation of settings and the future societies*. San Francisco, CA: Josey-Bass, Brookline Books.

Sawyer, J., & Brannock, D. (1990). Internalized dominance. *Angles*. Vancouver, British Columbia, Lavender Publishing Society. Winter

Seldes, G. (1985). *The great thoughts*. New York: Balantine Books.

Shelton, C., & Lipton, R. (1983). An alternative employment model. *Mental Retardation*, 33(2).

Skrtic, T. (1986). The crisis in special education knowledge: A perspective on perspective. *Focus on Exceptional Children* Vol. 18, No. 7.

Strong, P. M. (1979). Sociological Imperialism and the profession of medicine: A critical exam of the thesis of medical imperialism. *Social Science and Medicine* 13 A 199-215.

Stubbins, J. (1977). *Social and psychological aspects of disability*. Baltimore: University Park Press.

Sussman, M. (Ed.) (1959). *Community structure and analysis*. Thomas Crowell Co.

Swift, H., & Swift, E. (1964). *Community groups and you*. New York: John Day Co.

Szekeres, S., Ylvisaker, M., & Cohen, S. (1987). A framework for cognitive rehabilitation therapy. In M. Ylvisaker, & E. Gobble (Eds.), *Community re-entry for head injured adults*. Boston: College Hill Press.

Taylor, S., Biklen, D., & Knoll, J. (1987). *Community integration for people with severe disabilities*. New York: Teachers College Press.

Taylor, S., Racino, J., Knoll, J., & Lutfiyya, Z. (1987). Down home: Community integration for people with the most severe disabilities. In S. Taylor, D. Biklen, & J. Knoll, (Eds.), *Community integration for people with severe disabilities*. New York: Teachers College Press.

Thompsen, I. V. (1984). Late outcome of very severe blunt head trauma: A 10-15 year second follow-up. *Journal of Neurology, Neurosurgery, and Psychiatry*, Vol. 47.

Tissen, J. (1990). Attitudes toward disability as a function of epistemology and information framework. University of WIndson, Unpublished Masters Thesis.

Vanier, J. (1973). *Followers of Jesus*. Toronto: Griffith Press.

Wachter, J., Fawber, H.. & Scott, M. (1987). Treatment aspects of vocational evaluation and placement for traumatically brain injured adults. In M. Ylvisaker & E. M. Gobble, (Eds.), *Community re-entry for head injured adults*. Boston: College Hill Press.

Warren, R., & Warren, D. (1979). *The neighborhood organizer's handbook*. Notre Dame, IN: University of Notre Dame.

Wehman, P. (1975). "Toward a social skills curriculum for developmentally disabled clients in vocational settings". *Rehabilitation Literature*, Vol. 11.

Wehman, P., Kregel, J., & Barcus, J. M., (1985). From school to work: A vocational transition model for handicapped students. *Exceptional Children*. Vol. 52.

Wehman, P., & Kreutzer, J. (1989). *Supported employment workshop*. Dallas Rehabilitation Institute, Dallas, TX.

Wehman, P., & Moon, M. S. (1988). *Vocational rehabilitation and supported employment*. Baltimore: Paul H. Brookes Publishing Company.

Wehman, P., Renzaglia, A. and Bates, P. (1985). *Functional living skills for moderately and severely handicapped individuals*. Austin, TX: PRO-ED.

White, D. (1986). Social validation. In F. Rusch (Ed.), *Competitive employment issues and strategies*. Baltimore: Paul H. Brookes Publishing Company.

Williams, J. (1987). *Eyes on the prize*. New York: Viking Press.

Wirth, A. G. (19183). *Productive work in industry and schools: Becoming persons again*. Lanham, MD: University Press of America.

Whyte, W. F. (1943). *Street corner society*. Chicago, IL: University of Chicago Press.

Wolfensberger, W. (1971). *Normalization*. Toronto: National Institute on Mental Retardation.

Wolfensberger, W. (1983). *PASSING*. Toronto: National Institute on Mental Retardation.

Wolfensberger, W. (1987). *The new genocide of handicapped and affected people*. Syracuse: Training Institute for Human Service Planning, Leadership and Change Agentry.

Wolfensberger, W. (1990) A most critical issue. *Life or Death*. Vol. 8 No. 1.

Zola, I. K. (1986). The medicalization of aging and disability: Problems and prospects. In C. Mahoney, C. Estes, & J. Heumann (Eds.), *Toward a unified agenda*. Berkeley: World Institute on Disability.

Index

Index

A

──────── **B** ────────

──────── **C** ────────

——— **D** ———

Role expectations, rehabilitation and, 24-29
Role stereotypes, rehabilitation and, 25-29

S

Sarason, Seymore, on settings of human services, 47, 48
Self-esteem, empowerment and, 94-96
Sensitivity, empowerment and, 122-123
Service provision vs. advocacy in disability movement, 34-35
Setting for human services, 51-53
Shopping centers as community gathering places, 185
"Sick role" in medical paradigm of human services, 63-64
Sickness role, 20-21
Skills, assessment of, in economic paradigm, 73-74
Staff of human services, 51
Stereotypes, role, rehabilitation and, 25-29
Super markets as community gathering places, 185-186
Supports
    development of, in interdependent paradigm, 99-100
    limited, in interdependent paradigm, 90-91
    supplemental, in achieving interdependence, 142-144
Sussmen, Martin, on definition of community, 176
System
    change in, in interdependent paradigm, 100-102
    as core of problem in interdependent paradigm, 91-93
Systems advocacy in achieving interdependence, 150-157. *See also* Advocacy

T

Taverns
    as community gathering places, 184
    in learning about community, 189
Taylor, Steve, on "continuum trap," 103
Teacher, dominance of, in educational paradigm, 69-70
Training in economic paradigm, 74-75

U

University, interdependent environment of, 199

V

Vocational rehabilitation counselors in economic paradigm, 77

W

Warren, D.
    on community types, 181
    on definition of community, 175
    on definition of neighborhood, 179
    on functions of community, 180

Readers are invited to contact
Al Condeluci at UCP of Pittsburgh
4638 Centre Avenue
Pittsburgh, PA 15213

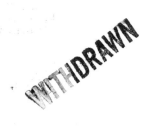